Structural Biology in Immunology

Structural Biology in Immunology

Structure/Function of Novel
Molecules of Immunologic Importance

Edited By

Chaim Putterman

David Cowburn

Steven Almo

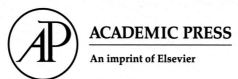

ACADEMIC PRESS
An imprint of Elsevier

Academic Press is an imprint of Elsevier
125 London Wall, London EC2Y 5AS, United Kingdom
525 B Street, Suite 1800, San Diego, CA 92101-4495, United States
50 Hampshire Street, 5th Floor, Cambridge, MA 02139, United States
The Boulevard, Langford Lane, Kidlington, Oxford OX5 1GB, United Kingdom

Notices
Knowledge and best practice in this field are constantly changing. As new research and experience
broaden our understanding, changes in research methods, professional practices, or medical
treatment may become necessary.

Practitioners and researchers must always rely on their own experience and knowledge in
evaluating and using any information, methods, compounds, or experiments described herein. In
using such information or methods they should be mindful of their own safety and the safety of
others, including parties for whom they have a professional responsibility.

To the fullest extent of the law, neither the Publisher nor the authors, contributors, or editors,
assume any liability for any injury and/or damage to persons or property as a matter of products
liability, negligence or otherwise, or from any use or operation of any methods, products,
instructions, or ideas contained in the material herein.

Library of Congress Cataloging-in-Publication Data
A catalog record for this book is available from the Library of Congress

British Library Cataloguing-in-Publication Data
A catalogue record for this book is available from the British Library

ISBN 978-0-12-803369-2

For information on all Academic Press publications
visit our website at https://www.elsevier.com/books-and-journals

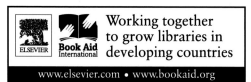

Working together
to grow libraries in
developing countries

www.elsevier.com • www.bookaid.org

Publisher: Mica Haley
Acquisition Editor: Linda Versteeg-buschman
Editorial Project Manager: Tracy Tufuga
Production Project Manager: Anusha Sambamoorthy
Cover Designer: Matthew Limbert

Typeset by SPi Global, India

Contents

Contributors   ix

1. **Organization of Immunological Synapses and Kinapses**
    Marco Fritzsche, Michael L. Dustin

    1.1 **Introduction**   2
    1.2 **Receptors and Ligands of the Immunological**
         Synapse and Kinapse   3
         1.2.1 T-cell Receptor and p^{Ag}MHC   3
         1.2.2 Adhesion Molecules   5
         1.2.3 Costimulatory and Checkpoint Receptors   7
         1.2.4 Nectins and Other Adhesion Receptors   9
         1.2.5 Coreceptors and Large Transmembrane Phosphatases   9
    1.3 **Phase-Like Behavior and Phase Separation in Signaling**   11
         1.3.1 Phase Separation in Adhesion Plane of Cell-Cell
                Interfaces   12
         1.3.2 Phase-Separated Lipid Domains in Plasma Membrane   13
         1.3.3 Phase Separation in Membrane Proximal Signaling   14
         1.3.4 Cytoskeletal Networks   14
    1.4 **Microvilli/Filopodia**   16
         1.4.1 Rosette-Shaped Actin Network   19
    1.5 **Synaptic Cleft Formation**   21
         1.5.1 Membrane Traffic to Maintain Signaling   21
         1.5.2 Extracellular Vesicles to Terminate Signaling and Relay
                Messages   22
         1.5.3 Directed Release of Effector Molecules Through Exocytosis   23
    1.6 **Conclusions**   24
         Acknowledgments   24
         References   24

2. **Principles of Protein Recognition by Small T-Cell**
    Adhesion Proteins and Costimulatory Receptors
    Shinji Ikemizu, Simon J. Davis

    2.1 **Introduction**   39
    2.2 **Cell-Cell Recognition and Adhesion: CD2 Family Proteins**   41

2.2.1	Rat sCD2 (1992)	42
2.2.2	Human sCD2 (1994)	46
2.2.3	The Role of Charged Residues in Ligand Binding by CD2 (1998)	48
2.2.4	CD58 d1 (1999)	50
2.2.5	CD48 d1 (2006)	52
2.3	**Cell-Cell Recognition and Costimulation: CD28 Family Proteins**	54
2.3.1	sB7-1 (2000)	56
2.3.2	sCTLA-4/sB7-1 Complex (2001)	59
2.3.3	sCD28/5.11A1 Antibody Fab (2005)	61
2.3.4	sCTLA-4 (2011)	64
2.3.5	sPD-1 (2013)	66
2.4	**Concluding Remarks**	69
	Acknowledgments	72
	References	72

3. Synthetic Antibody Engineering: Concepts and Applications

Jonathan R. Lai, Gang Chen, Sachdev S. Sidhu

3.1	**Introduction**	81
3.2	**Immunoglobulin Structure and Function**	83
3.3	**Engineering Phage-Displayed Antibody Libraries**	85
3.4	**Applications**	90
3.4.1	Engineering of Conformation-Specific Antibodies	90
3.4.2	Engineering of Cross-Reactive Antibodies	92
3.4.3	Engineering of Antibodies Specific for Point-Mutants and PTMs	94
3.5	**Conclusions**	96
	References	96

4. Natural Killer Cell Receptors

Sneha Rangarajan, Roy A. Mariuzza

4.1	**Introduction**	101
4.2	**MHC-I Recognition by Ly49 Receptors**	102
4.3	**Ly49 Receptors Interact With MHC-I in *Trans* and *Cis***	104
4.4	**Ly49A's Recognition of a Viral Immunoevasin**	105
4.5	**Recognition of MHC-I by KIR Receptors**	106
4.6	**Recognition of MHC-I by LILRs**	108
4.7	**LILR Recognition of the Viral Immunoevasin UL18**	110
4.8	**Natural Cytotoxicity Receptors**	110
4.9	**Ligand Binding by NKG2D**	112
4.10	**HLA-E Recognition by NKG2/CD94**	114
4.11	**Recognition of Cadherins by KLRG1**	114
4.12	**C-type Lectin-like Receptor-Ligand Pairs in the NK Gene Complex**	115

4.13 Perspective   117
References   117

5. **Structure-Function in Antibodies to
Double-Stranded DNA**
Yumin Xia, Ertan Eryilmaz, David Cowburn, Chaim Putterman

5.1 Anti-dsDNA Antibodies Are Pivotal in the Pathogenesis
of Lupus Erythematosus   127
5.2 The Basic Features of Antigen Recognition by Anti-dsDNA
Antibodies   129
5.3 The Constant Regions Contribute to Antigenic
Specificity and Renal Pathogenicity of Anti-dsDNA
Antibodies   130
5.4 The Structure of Anti-dsDNA Antibodies   131
5.5 Catalytic Properties of Anti-dsDNA Antibodies   134
5.6 DNA-Mimicking Peptides Bound by Anti-dsDNA
Antibodies   136
5.7 Development of Novel Therapeutic Approaches
Targeting Anti-dsDNA Antibodies In Vivo   138
References   140

6. **The Role of the Constant Region in Antibody-Antigen
Interactions: Redefining the Modular Model of
Immunoglobulin Structure**
Anthony Bowen, Arturo Casadevall

6.1 Introduction   145
6.2 Immunoglobulin Structure   146
6.3 The Modular Antibody Model   151
6.4 Evidence for Intramolecular Signaling Upon Antigen Binding   154
6.5 Constant Region Modulation of Antibody Properties   157
6.6 Concluding Remarks   163
References   163

Index   171

Contributors

Numbers in parentheses indicate the pages on which the authors' contributions begin.

Anthony Bowen (145), Albert Einstein College of Medicine, New York, NY, United States

Arturo Casadevall (145), Johns Hopkins Bloomberg School of Public Health, Baltimore, MD, United States

Gang Chen (81), University of Toronto, Toronto, ON, Canada

David Cowburn (127), Albert Einstein College of Medicine, New York, NY, United States

Simon J. Davis (39), University of Oxford, Oxford, United Kingdom

Michael L. Dustin (1), Kennedy Institute of Rheumatology, Oxford, United Kingdom; New York University School of Medicine, New York, NY, United States

Ertan Eryilmaz (127), Albert Einstein College of Medicine, New York, NY, United States

Marco Fritzsche (1), Kennedy Institute of Rheumatology; Weatherall Institute of Molecular Medicine, University of Oxford, Oxford, United Kingdom

Shinji Ikemizu (39), Kumamoto University, Kumamoto, Japan

Jonathan R. Lai (81), Albert Einstein College of Medicine, Bronx, NY, United States

Roy A. Mariuzza (101), University of Maryland Institute for Bioscience and Biotechnology Research, Rockville; University of Maryland, College Park, MD, United States

Chaim Putterman (127), Albert Einstein College of Medicine and Montefiore Medical Center, Bronx, NY, United States

Sneha Rangarajan (101), University of Maryland Institute for Bioscience and Biotechnology Research, Rockville; University of Maryland, College Park, MD, United States

Sachdev S. Sidhu (81), University of Toronto, Toronto, ON, Canada

Yumin Xia (127), Albert Einstein College of Medicine, New York, NY, United States

Chapter 1

Organization of Immunological Synapses and Kinapses

Marco Fritzsche*,†, Michael L. Dustin*,‡

*Kennedy Institute of Rheumatology, Oxford, United Kingdom, †Weatherall Institute of Molecular Medicine, University of Oxford, Oxford, United Kingdom, ‡New York University School of Medicine, New York, NY, United States

ABBREVIATIONS

Ag	antigen
Arp	actin-related protein
CD(#)	cluster of differentiation (1,2,3…)
CRTAM	class-I MHC-restricted T-cell-associated molecule
CSK	C-terminal Src kinase
CTLA-4	cytotoxic T lymphocyte antigen-4
DC	dendritic cell
ICAM(#)	intercellular adhesion molecule-(1,2,3…)
ICOS(L)	inducible T-cell costimulator (ligand)
ITAM	immunotyrosine activation motif
LAT	linker of activated T cells
LFA-(#)	lymphocyte function associated-(1,2,3)
(p)MHC	(peptide) major histocompatibility complex
PD-1	programmed cell death-1
SH(#)	Src homology domain (1,2,3)
SIM	structured illumination microscopy
SLAM	signaling lymphocyte activation molecule
SLB	supported lipid bilayer
(c,p,d)SMAC	(central, peripheral, distal) supramolecular activation cluster
STED	stimulated excitation depletion
TCR	T-cell antigen receptor
(e)TIRF(M)	(extended) total internal reflection fluorescence (microscopy)
VASP	vasodilator-stimulated phosphoprotein
WASp	Wiscott Aldrich syndrome protein
ZAP-70	TCR zeta-associated protein of 70 kili-Daltons

Structural Biology in Immunology. https://doi.org/10.1016/B978-0-12-803369-2.00001-2

1.1 INTRODUCTION

Immunological synapses are stable adhesive junctions formed by immune cells for priming of immune responses and effector function.[1] The archetype is based on radially symmetric junctions formed by helper or cytotoxic T cells, with B cells as antigen-presenting cells in which concentric zones referred to as supramolecular activation clusters (SMACs) can be resolved by wide-field microscopy in vitro and in vivo.[2,3] The most important function of the immunological synapses is directed secretion of regulatory signals in the form of proteins and vesicles between immune cells, and also killing of pathogens in the context of innate immune recognition (,[4–7] p. 5140). Immunological synapses are formed by T cells, innate lymphoid cells, B cells, mast cells, neutrophils, macrophages (phagocytic synapse), and likely others.[5,7–10] The key common denominator is that specificity is driven by receptors that couple to nonreceptor tyrosine kinases, often through immunotyrosine activation motifs in the cytoplasmic domain.[11] The T-cell antigen receptor (TCR) is the relevant receptor for T cells,[12] which will be the major focus of this chapter.

The formation of the archetypal T-cell immunological synapse can also be reconstituted with supported lipid bilayers (SLBs) containing major histocompatibility complex (MHC) proteins with bound agonist peptides ($p^{Ag}MHC$) and the adhesion molecule intercellular adhesion molecule-1 (ICAM-1, CD54) in which SMACs form in a time-dependent manner.[10] The two major SMACs are the central SMAC (cSMAC), which is enriched in T-cell receptors (TCRs), $p^{Ag}MHC$, and some costimulatory receptors such as CD28, and the peripheral SMAC (pSMAC) that is enriched in the integrin lymphocyte function associated 1 (LFA-1, CD11a) and ICAM-1[2] (Fig. 1.1A). Subsequently, Freiberg et al. defined the distal SMAC (dSMAC) as a ring outside the pSMAC enriched in CD45 and dynamic filamentous actin (F-actin).[13,14] Some aspects of immunological synapse formation can also be reconstituted with glass substrates coated with anti-CD3 antibodies to trigger TCR signals and other surface treatments, such as poly-L-lysine or serum attachment factors (fibronectin, vitronectin, etc.) that provide an adhesion component.[15,16] In the absence of this adhesion component, anti-CD3 elicits actin-rich protrusions that push the cell away from the anti-CD3-coated surface.[17,18] We will incorporate data from cell-cell systems and model substrates to generate a current picture and trajectory for future questions.

Stability of the immunological synapse depends on its symmetry. Breaking of the symmetry of the immunological synapse leads to a migratory junction defined as a kinapse, which appears to be an important mode of T-cell interaction with, for example, dendritic cells (DCs) and germinal center B cells in vivo[10,13,19–23] (Fig. 1.1B). Kinapse formation may lead to "multifocal synapses" observed in T-DC interactions in vitro and in vivo.[24,25] The immunological synapse and kinapse share signaling elements, referred to as microclusters, which are formed by both the TCR and LFA-1.[26–29] While the formation of

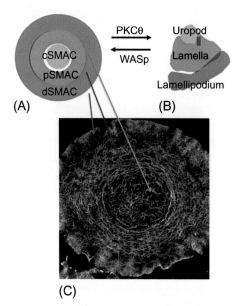

FIG. 1.1   Supramolecular activation clusters in synapse and kinapse. (A) Schematic view of the Kupferian SMACs as originally defined in immunological synapse and remapped to kinapse. Note that the cSMAC, pSMAC, and dSMAC (defined in text) are related to structures in kinapse by symmetry breaking. Based on Sims et al.[13] the activity of PKC-θ favors kinapse whereas the activity of WASp favors synapse. (B) eTIRF-SIM image of F-actin network in Jurkat T cell. The regions of the rosette-like network that correspond to the SMACs are indicated. See text for further discussion of the limitations of these assignments.

microclusters likely has some aspects driven by the biophysics of receptor-ligand-driven self-assembly in the interface, most aspects of immunological synapse and kinapse formation and maturation are dependent upon intact F-actin cytoskeleton and later stages of synapse maturation are regulated by microtubules.[30–32] The chapter will build a structural model for the immunological synapse beginning with some major classes of receptors and then moving to the underlying cytoskeletal networks and important issues of membrane topology.

1.2   RECEPTORS AND LIGANDS OF THE IMMUNOLOGICAL SYNAPSE AND KINAPSE

1.2.1   T-cell Receptor and p^{Ag}MHC

There are two known TCR heterodimers—αβ and γδ—that are expressed on distinct subsets of T cells.[12] The classical adaptive T-cell subsets use the αβ TCR, whereas subsets of tissue-resident T cells use the γδ TCR.[33] Most γδ T cells and a small subset of αβ T cells are innate like, meaning that they use stereotypical rearrangements to generate largely invariant receptors for conserved ligands that are often presented on nonclassical MHC-like proteins. For example, the so-called natural killer T cells use invariant αβ TCR to recognize glycolipids bound to CD1d, which has a structure similar to MHC class I, but possesses a binding groove adapted for the recognition of glycolipids.[34] Mucosal-associated invariant T cells recognize microbial metabolites presented on MHC-related protein.[35] This chapter focuses on the majority of αβ T cells that use MHC class I or class II proteins as ligands in combinations with short peptides. Each of these αβ T cells expresses one TCR that binds weakly to self-peptide (p^{self})-MHC based on thymic selection and has the potential to bind a variety of p^{Ag}MHC.[36] Since each TCR is generated through multiple recombination events involving germline V, (D), and J segments with random addition of base pairs during joining, there is huge diversity of these weakly self-reactive TCR in the "naïve" repertoire that are selected for expansion and conversion into memory T cells over the life of an individual. The interaction of TCR with p^{self}–MHC is challenging to measure physically using the available methods, but in solution have dissociation constants on the order of 100 μM to >1 mM,[37,38] yet these interactions are essential for thymic selection during development and appear to influence mature T cells continuously.[39] The interactions of TCR with p^{Ag}MHC typically have Kd in the range of 100 nM–10 μM.[38] All individuals seem to harbor some higher affinity p^{self}-MHC-specific T cells that often take on suppressive roles as regulatory T cells (Treg),[40] but can also be recruited into anti-pathogen responses and contribute to autoimmune diseases.[41,42]

The description of the interaction of TCR with pMHC through solution affinity is an imperfect predictor of function,[43] as the receptor system exclusively operates in an interface between two biological membranes. This introduces two key features. First, in order for the TCR to interact with pMHC, the two membranes need to be separated by <15 nm, with measurements from electron microscopy suggesting ~13 nm as the average intermembrane distance generated by large numbers of these interactions.[44] The other aspect is that due to the cytoskeletal dynamics that we will describe, the interactions are subjected to physical forces.[10,15,45,46] There are two well-described bond types for force-bearing interactions in biology—slip bonds in which the off-rate increases with force in the pN range, and catch bonds, where the bond off-rate decreases at an optimal force.[47] It has been shown by two independent methods, biomolecular force probe and laser trap, that TCR-p^{Ag}MHC interactions are catch bonds with a force optimum around 10 pN.[48,49] This force requirement is a key feature that distinguishes the immature T cell selecting p^{self}-MHC interactions, which form slip binds, from the mature T-cell-activating p^{Ag}MHC, which form catch bonds.[49] However, recent studies suggest that the pre-TCR, expressed by thymocytes following rearrangement of the TCR β subunit, can also form catch bonds with p^{self}-MHC complexes.[50] The structural features that distinguish the slip and catch bonds are not known, but laser trap measurements suggest that the catch bond undergoes a conformational transition that extends the complex by 10 nm, which is 66% of the apparent length of the unstrained complex.[48]

This suggests significant unfolding of β-sheet structures as part of the force-dependent transition. There is some evidence that the tangential orientation of force relative to the T-cell surface is more effective than normal orientation.[51,52] Possible explanations for this are discussed in the context of functions of TCR microclusters.

1.2.2 Adhesion Molecules

T cells are sensitive to a single pMHC and this can be accomplished in part because of the activity of adhesion molecules.[53,54] We will define adhesion molecules as surface receptors that are present in high copy number (on the order of 100,000 molecules) on both the T cell and the antigen-presenting cell. This high expression level allows adhesion molecules to contribute to the generation of the close contacts needed for TCR to reach the pMHC on the surface of the APC. There are two general adhesion molecules in human T cells that are extensively utilized in cell-cell interactions: the integrin family member LFA-1 and the signaling lymphocyte activation molecule (SLAM) family member CD2.[53] Other integrins and other SLAM family members participate in different settings, but we will focus on these as the best-studied paradigms.

Integrins are large cell surface heterodimers that interact with ligands in a divalent cation and in an energy-dependent manner. The large extracellular domains have an N-terminal globular domain made up of large (α) and small (β) subunits that bind to ligand with high or low affinity depending upon the conformation.[55] The globular domain is connected to the two transmembrane domains by 15 nm stalks. The small cytoplasmic domains interact with a number of regulatory factors, most importantly the F-actin linker talin and the regulatory protein kindlin 3.[56] Genetic deficiency of the β subunit of LFA-1 (referred to as β2 or CD18) or kindling 3 leads to leukocyte adhesion deficiency diseases (types I and III, respectively) that particularly impact specific innate cellular functions involved in protection from bacterial infection, and quantitatively impair aspects of adaptive immunity.[56,57] Antibodies against LFA-1 were used in the treatment of autoimmune diseases including psoriasis until adverse events including fatal viral infections forced their removal from the market.[58,59] This experience underscores the great importance of adhesion molecules in many aspects of the immune response, including the homing of cells through interactions with endothelial cells, such that global inhibition of a major adhesion molecule has significant risks. LFA-1 is well characterized structurally with crystal structures of its ligand-binding domain without and with the relevant immunoglobulin (Ig)-like domain from the ligand ICAM-1.[60] There is also extensive information about LFA-1 conformations from electron microscopy studies.[61] Like other integrins, LFA-1 exists in low affinity form, where the stalks are bent to bring the ligand-binding domain very close to the T-cell membrane. Activation of the molecules by separation of the cytoplasmic domains results in extension so that the ligand-binding site projects to ~20 nm from the membrane, and together with the ~14 nm length of ICAM-1 (which has an L-shaped molecule with 5 Ig-like domains), the LFA-1-ICAM-1 interaction could span up to 34 nm between membranes.[62] However, like the TCR, LFA-1 may subjected to mechanical forces that are tangential to the T-cell membrane during synapse or kinapse formation, such that the actual intermembrane distance may be smaller due to the lateral pulling against ICAM-1 that is anchored to the cytoskeleton.[63] In addition to ICAM-1, human LFA-1 binding to several other ligands, the most important of which is the 2 Ig-like domain ICAM-2.[64] It is not clear if interaction with this shorter ligand generates different intermembrane spacing or clustering of LFA-1. Generally, TCR-pMHC interactions segregate laterally from LFA-1-ICAM-1 interaction. The precise mechanism by which LFA-1-ICAM-1 interactions promote TCR-pMHC interactions is not entirely clear, but it may involve generating force-resistant adhesion against which the cell can push TCR-rich projections against the substrate (see the section on scanning interactions).[10,65,66]

CD2 continuously diffuses into the T-cell membrane and binds to CD58 (T11, LFA-2, sheep erythrocyte receptor), a ligand expressed on all cells, even erythrocytes.[67] CD2 and CD58 are both members of the SLAM subfamily of the Ig-superfamily, which resides in a cluster on chromosome 1 in the mouse and human. CD2 and CD58 bind to each other with a Kd of ~ 1 μM and the interaction dissociates very rapidly with a koff of $>7 s^{-1}$.[68] A crystal structure exists for human CD2 interacting with CD58, which provides a detailed structural basis of its adhesive function.[69] In rodents, the major CD2 ligand is CD48, which also exists in humans as a distinct gene from CD58. Mice lack a homologue of CD58. In both mouse and human, CD48 is a ligand for the 2B4 receptor (CD244), an activating receptor highly expressed on natural killer cells, but also activated T cells.[70] Thus, in rodents CD2 and 2B4 may compete for CD48 and the affinity is mouse CD2 for the mouse CD48 is 10-fold lower than for human CD2 and CD58.[71] Nonetheless, mouse CD2 contributes to T-cell activation in a nonredundant manner.[53,72] The distinct contributions of CD2 likely arise from its distinct mode of adhesion and from its highly conserved cytoplasmic domain. In contrast to the situation with integrins, adhesion mediated by CD2 interactions with CD58 is neither divalent cation nor energy dependent. Like the TCR-pMHC, it spans an apparent distance between membranes of ~15 nm with a measured intermembrane distance of 13 nm.[73,74] The CD2-CD58 interaction is the first adhesion system for which a 2D affinity, as defined by Bell,[75] was measured,[76] partly because its mode of adhesion is highly amenable to this type of analysis. The 2D Kd is $~1 \mu m^{-2}$ indicating a highly efficient assembly process that positions the binding sites in a very small volume, with an axial dimension of ~5 nm, and a lateral dimension of micrometers.[77] An immunological synapse has an interaction area of ~50 μm². This means that the ~10,000 CD2 and CD58 molecules in the interface when the cells come into contact are at an effective concentration of 66 μM, which exceeds the three-dimensional (3D) Kd for mouse or human CD2 for its ligand.[71] While there are some barriers to forming such close contacts between cells,[78] once the close contact is nucleated this adhesion system is very efficient, but at the same time very dynamic, such that the CD2-CD58 interaction turns over rapidly and does not impede cell migration. As CD2-CD58 interactions span the same distance at the TCR-pMHC, it is not surprising that the presence of CD2-ligand interactions increases the sensitivity of TCR for p^{Ag}MHC.[72] In fact, increasing the size of CD48 to produce a mismatch with the TCR-pMHC dimensions profoundly inhibits T-cell detection of pMHC on APCs expressing the extended CD48 molecules.[79] There are autoimmune disease risk alleles associated with CD2 and CD58, and recently, a CD2 signaling signature was associated with increased severity of autoimmune diseases.[80] CD2 has a long cytoplasmic domain with five polyproline motifs that interact with SH3 domains of Fyn and an adapter protein referred to as CD2-associated protein.[81] Under specific cross-linking conditions CD2 ligation alone can be strongly mitogenic for T cells,[82] but there is no known physiological signaling mode that fully exploits this strong, antigen-independent activation.[83] The CD2 cytoplasmic domain lacks any tyrosine residues and thus may utilize the regulatory mechanisms based on tyrosine phosphatase recruitment.

The SLAM family contains a number of other receptors most of which are homophilic (self-binding) and have cytoplasmic domains that bind to SH2D1A and B, which are single SH2 domain adapters that interact with the Src family kinase Fyn.[84] SH2D1A mutations result in X-link lymphoproliferative disease 1, which is characterized by defects in the regulation of myeloid cells and hypogammaglobulinemia due to defects in T-cell help for B cells.[85] In this situation, the tyrosine in the cytoplasmic domain of most SLAM family members (excluding CD2, 2B4, and CD48) recruits the tyrosine phosphatase SHP2 leading to a dominant inhibitory effect.[86] The normal function of SLAM family members is in adhesion, likely in conjunction with CD2-CD58/CD48 and LFA-1-ICAM-1 interactions. Another nonredundant function of SLAM family members and SAP is in the selection of NKT cells in the thymus.[87] CD1d is expressed on other thymocytes and positive selection and expansion of NKT cells is mediated by thymocyte-thymocyte interactions that require SLAM family members and the Fyn kinase that is recruited to engage SLAM receptors by SH2D1A. The relevant SLAM family members for T-B and NKT selection include CD84, CD150, CD229, and CD352.[88] Crystal structures for CD84, CD150, and CD229 reveal homophilic interactions with overall similar to the CD2-CD58 heterophilic interactions that would likely operate with a similar intermembrane spacing to TCR-pMHC. In general, the SLAM family members play an important role in lymphocyte-lymphocyte interactions.[89]

1.2.3   Costimulatory and Checkpoint Receptors

Costimulatory receptors act in concert with TCR signals to shift T cells from tolerogenic signaling with TCR engagement only to immunogenic signaling that promotes survival and differentiation of T cells into effector and memory T cells.

CD28 is the most well-known costimulatory molecule; CD28 is a dimeric member of the Ig superfamily that interacts with two ligands, CD80 and CD86 (also referred to as B7-1 and B7-2, respectively).[90] A defining characteristic of the costimulatory systems is that the receptors are typically expressed at >10-fold lower levels than adhesion molecules, making them dependent on TCR microcluster formation for engagement.[91] The levels of CD80 and CD86 are tightly regulated and are particularly unregulated on mature DC and activated B cells.[90] Two inhibitory or "checkpoint" receptors regulate CD28 signaling, cytotoxic T lymphocyte antigen-4 (CTLA-4, CD152), and programmed death-1 (PD-1, CD279). CTLA-4 is expressed during T-cell activation and competes with CD28 for binding to CD80 and CD86 and is also used by Treg to strip these molecules off of the surface of antigen-presenting cells, thus limiting CD28-mediated costimulation.[92] PD-1 utilizes a different strategy to inhibit CD28 signals. PD-1 co-clusters with TCR and CD28 in microclusters and recruits a SH2 domain-containing phosphatase SHP2 that dephosphorylates tyrosines in the cytoplasmic domain of CD28, limiting both PKC-θ-mediated NF-κB activation and phosphatidylinositol 3-kinase activation by CD28.[93] PD-1 is expressed at low levels during the activation of T cells, but is further upregulated by chronic antigen exposure, such as that happens in chronic viral infections. The ligands for PD-1, PDL1 (CD274), and PDL2 (CD273) are widely expressed on myeloid and stromal cells, and also on activated T cells.[94] The high expression of PDL1 on tumor cells may blunt the activation of tumor-infiltrating lymphocytes, although recent studies suggest that the major effect of PD-1 blockade in therapy for chronic viral infection and cancer is the CD28-dependent expansion of antigen-specific T cells, which would generally be thought to occur in draining lymph nodes rather that in tissue sites or tumors.[95] Of the current exciting checkpoint blockade therapies, anti-PD-1 antibodies appear to have the best balance of efficacy and low toxicity.[96]

CD28 is constitutively expressed on T cells and loss of CD28 expression is a signature of senescence, a state of low fitness for survival, and low capacity for cell division.[97] The other major constitutively expressed costimulatory receptor is CD27, a member of the tumor necrosis factor receptor family that binds to the ligand CD70, which is a member of the TNF family. CD27 is particularly highly expressed on developing T and B cells and the ligand, CD70, is highly expressed on thymic epithelial cells. Interestingly, CD27 is also lost on senescent T cells. It has been demonstrated that CD70 is upregulated on B cells infected with EBV and an inherited deficiency of CD27 or CD70 in humans leads to Epstein-Barr virus (EBV) infection.[98]

There are a number of inducible co-stimulatory receptors including the inducible T-cell co-stimulator (ICOS, CD278) and several TNFR family members including CD357, CD137, and CD134. ICOS plays an important role in T cell help for B cells by interacting with ICOS ligand (CD275) expressed on B cells.[99] ICOS is a potent inducer of phosphatidylinositol 3-kinase activity and this may be related to its impact on migration and interactions. Recently, we have shown that ICOS-ligand (ICOSL, CD275) induced by B cells by dopamine signaling enhances the delivery of CD40L (CD154) to the helper T-cell immunological synapse.[100] CD40 is a TNF receptor family member on antigen-presenting cells that provides critical activating signals for DC maturation and B-cell activation/differentiation.[101] The ligand for CD357 is highly expressed on skin-resident DCs called Langerhan's cells and on red pulp macrophages in the spleen[102]; however, its complete absence on circulating immune cells has resulting in its failure to be identified in the CD nomenclature system. CD134 deficiency results in classical Kaposi's sarcoma, a virally induced tumor of endothelial cells.[103] The ligand for CD134, CD252 is also associated with atherosclerosis risk and is expressed on hematopoietic progenitors, activated mast cells, and activated endothelial cells. CD137 is expressed early in CD8 T-cell activation and also on a variety of myeloid cells types and stromal cells. The ligand is more restricted with high expression in activated macrophages, Langerhan's cells, liver DCs, and some stromal cell types in lymph nodes (Podoplanin and CD31 negative subset) and medullary thymic epithelial cells. Signaling motifs taken from CD137 have proven particularly useful in engineering T cells with long-term persistence in vivo.[104]

1.2.4   Nectins and Other Adhesion Receptors

Another family of Ig-like adhesion molecules on immune cells are the nectins. These receptors participate in a broad range of homophilic and heterophilic interactions, and less is known about their function in immune response.[105] One of these receptors, class-I MHC-restricted T-cell-associated molecule (CRTAM, CD355), is associated with a subset of CD4 T cells that elaborate a cytotoxic program.[106] Furthermore, forced CRTAM expression in CRTAM-negative CD4 T cells imposed a cytotoxic program on these cells, suggesting that CRTAM is not only a subset marker, but is a functional receptor that activates this program, potentially through homophilic or heterophilic interactions during priming. Thus, there may be a wealth of additional regulation that emerges when this large group of surface receptors is more fully studied. T cells also express a number of receptors with C-type lectin domains, which have activating and co-stimulatory functions in subsets of activated T cells. Generally, it has been found that despite having "lectin" domains, these proteins are involved in protein-protein recognition. L-selectin (CD62L), which is critical for interaction with glycan ligands on endothelial cells during T-cell trafficking has also been implicated in other roles within tissues.[107]

1.2.5   Coreceptors and Large Transmembrane Phosphatases

The TCR signals via recruitment of nonreceptor tyrosine kinases lymphocyte kinase (Lck) and zeta-associated kinase of 70 kDa (ZAP-70) to the receptor.[11] Lck is associated with the inner leaflet of the plasma membrane via N-terminal lipid modifications and associates with CD4 and CD8 coreceptors, which interact with MHC class II and class I, respectively. During thymic development, CD4 and CD8 double-positive thymocytes that have a weak interaction with either p^{self}-MHC class I or II downregulate CD8 for a period of time. If they lose signaling during this period, meaning that p^{self}-MHC class I was the ligand of the TCR, they are instructed to reexpress CD8 and silence CD4 transcription.[108] If signaling is not lost during this period, that is, when the p^{self}-MHC class II is engaging the TCR, the cells maintain expression of CD4 and silence CD8. Thus, the immature T cell chooses which type of coreceptor to express through an instructive process. The interaction of CD4 with MHC class II is of extremely low affinity, and a 2D affinity of $5000\,\mu m^{-2}$ was measured for this interaction.[109] It has been proposed that additional interactions mediated by Lck in the context of the TCR ligand by p^{Ag}MHC will stabilize the signaling complex such that the CD4 interaction with MHC class II only needs to initiate the interaction, but then will rapidly leave unless phosphorylation is initiated.[110] The regulation of Lck activity, whether or not is bound to the coreceptor, is critical for forming this successful complex.

Lck activity is determined by autophosphorylation of its activation loop, but this process is controlled by two intramolecular interactions. Lck, like other Src family kinases, has a unique N-terminal region (in this case used to interact with the membrane and with coreceptors), an SH3 domain (polyproline binding), an SH2 domain (phosphotyrosine binding), and the SH1 domain (kinase).[111] The inactive form of Lck is favored when the C-terminal inhibitory tyrosine (Y505 in Lck) is phosphorylated by the C-terminal Src kinase (CSK).[112] CSK is recruited to the membrane via its SH2 domain, which binds sites in multiple transmembrane adapter proteins that are phosphorylated by active Lck and other Src family kinases.[113] This results in intramolecular interactions of the SH2 domain with the C-terminal phosphotyrosine. An additional intramolecular interaction between the SH3 domain with a connecting peptide between the SH2 and kinase domains also contributes to keeping Lck in an inactive state. Activation of the Lck is favored when Y505 is dephosphorylated by the large transmembrane tyrosine phosphatase CD45.[114] Competing ligands for the SH2 and SH3 domains can also promote activation, but the intramolecular interaction of the SH2 and the pY505 is so efficient that T cells without CD45 cannot be activated. However, CD45 is a relatively promiscuous tyrosine phosphatase and can also dephosphorylate the activation loop and other targets of Lck and ZAP-70.[93] Once active Lck is recruited to the TCR, it phosphorylates the immunotyrosine activation motifs of the TCR/CD3 complex cytoplasmic domains, of which there are 10 motifs with 2 tyrosines each and then recruits ZAP-70. The ITAM binding conformation of ZAP-70 is further stabilized by additional Lck-mediated phosphorylations within ZAP-70. The recruited ZAP-70 then transphosphorylates each other's activation loops, which increases the kinase activity and allows phosphorylation of tyrosine motifs in the transmembrane adapter protein called linker of activated T cells (LAT).[115] LAT has four sites that are phosphorylated by ZAP-70 and recruits additional adapters and the critical enzyme phospholipase C-γ which cleaves phosphatidylinositol-4,5-bis phosphate to generate diacylglycerol and inositol-1,4,5-trisphosphate leading to the activation of RAS-GRP, PKC-θ, and calcium release from intracellular stores.[116] A parallel process, also dependent on ITAM phosphorylation, recruits Vav, which mediates an F-actin remodeling-dependent activation of Notch receptors that also contribute to the T-cell transcriptional response, particularly with regard to proliferation.[117] While CD45 is important for maintaining active Lck, it can also inhibit this cascade if fully unchecked. The large extracellular domain of CD45 provides one mechanism for reducing CD45 density in regions of the immunological synapse where TCR binds pMHC.[46,118]

The structure of the extracellular domain of CD45 has recently been determined and it is clear that its four fibronectin type III repeats, which are similar to Ig domains, for a single rigid structure with a length of 15.2 nm.[119] The effective bulk of the extracellular domain is also increased by an S/T-rich N-terminal extension, which is longest in naïve T cells and shorter in memory T cells, due to alternative splicing. Thus, the CD45 extracellular domain is too large to fit into the 13 nm gap between membranes at sites of TCR-pMHC interaction, which leads to a partial and highly localized exclusion. This local exclusion provides an effective compromise between CD45's positive role in activating LCK and its negative role in blocking the tyrosine kinase cascade needed for signaling. Importantly, the CD2-CD58/48 interactions also exclude CD45 when it operates in an antigen-independent manner and there is a weak, but measurable calcium signal associated with this process, but this does not result in T-cell activation.[83] The lack of strong signaling on CD2 engagement is probably because TCR is also weakly excluded from these close contacts and because CSK will inactivate Lck whenever its diffusion distance from CD45 exceeds the half-time for CSK phosphorylation of Lck on Y505.[120] This phenomenon provides a check against excessive TCR signaling in large close contacts formed by adhesion molecules like CD2-CD58. We will discuss it further in the context of microclusters.

With these elements in mind, we think about higher-order structures in the immunological synapse and how they contribute to the overall function of the immunological synapse. The next level building block is supramolecular assemblies that are proximal to the TCR/co-stimulation and adhesion microclusters.

1.3 PHASE-LIKE BEHAVIOR AND PHASE SEPARATION IN SIGNALING

Phase separation has long been studied in biology. Classical phases of matter such as gas, liquid, and solid can be combined and will form interfaces that exchange components and interconvert between steady states under critical conditions.[121] In biology, a particularly interesting mode of phase separation involves liquid-liquid phases where weak interactions of solutes in a bulk solvent reach critical concentrations to form physical compartments with distant compositions that readily exchange components across a discrete boundary.[121,122] The boundaries in liquid-liquid systems will tend to minimize line tension leading to spherical shapes in 3D and circles in two-dimensional (2D) systems. The liquid nature of the phases means that they may undergo fusion and fission with application of appropriate external forces and they will relax to the spherical/circular shape. Some phases are miscible based on shared interactions or constraints, whereas others are immiscible, providing a basis for sorting and mixing in highly dynamic and reversible systems. We will consider three examples of phase-like behavior in the immunological synapse: 2D adhesion, 2D membrane bilayer composition, and 3D signaling complexes. We will then consider how these phases interact with the cortical actin network,[123] which are hydrated solids.

1.3.1 Phase Separation in Adhesion Plane of Cell-Cell Interfaces

The energy released through interactions of hundreds or thousands of low-affinity, fast dissociating adhesion molecules in the interface between cells may be utilized to sort the interacting proteins into lateral domains and also to influence the lateral positioning of other proteins, such as CD45, based on steric and entropic effects. As mentioned earlier, the CD2-CD58 interaction is an excellent example of an adhesion system that operates through many low-affinity, short-lived interactions. Going back to the early studies on CD2-CD58 interactions in the interface of live T cells and SLBs, there are many characteristics of the adhesion interfaces that are phase like. A CD2-positive T cell interacting with an SLB containing CD58 will first nucleate a number of small clusters that likely reflect projections from the cell that make first contact with the SLB and nucleate CD2-CD58 interactions that then glow progressively.[76,124] At 24°C, T cells have relatively low motility and polarity such that these domains are free to encounter and fuse with each other as they grow and the most peripheral projections that form islands of interaction outside the growing central contact area are free to fuse with it when they come close to each other or to the central adhesion domain. The result is a near perfect circular adhesion zone that will remain at this steady state for many hours.[76] When SLB containing CD58 and ICAM-1 are utilized the CD2-CD58 and LFA-1-ICAM1 interactions segregate systematically with sharp boundaries, which are also observed in cell-cell interfaces.[125] Experiments that extend pMHC or CD48 (as a ligand for mouse CD2) by two or three Ig-like domains predicted that each Ig-like domain would add 4 nm to the intermembrane distance, but measurements by electron microscopy in cell-cell or cell-SLB interfaces found that each Ig-like domain added only 1 nm to the intermembrane separation, such that increasing the length of the molecules seems to further increase the degree of tilting of the proteins in the interface.[74] Furthermore, the apparent 2D affinity was decreased by ~10-fold by addition of two or three Ig-like domains, suggesting that the binding sites were moving through a much large volume to encounter each other compared with the situation with the natural two Ig-like domain SLAM family scaffold.

The physical basis of protein exclusion based on the extracellular domain size has been modeled using tandem fluorescent proteins at the interface between giant unilamellar vesicles (GUVs) or between GUV and SLB.[126] This model exploited the weak interaction of natural green fluorescent protein dimers to mediate adhesion between GUV and then addition of spacer modules based on a dark (nonfluorescent) mCherry construct to generate different intermembrane separations. Tandem fluorescent mCherry constructs that have no interaction with the other elements were then imaged to determine how their size in relation to the adhesion constructs impacted exclusion from contact areas. Interestingly, partial exclusion (~50% of maximal) was observed when the noninteracting protein size matched the predicted intermembrane separation and then rapidly reached maximal levels (~80%) when the noninteracting protein was just one module larger than the predicted intermembrane separation and there was no exclusion when the noninteracting proteins were one module shorter than that of intermembrane separation. Thus, even though the structured domain of CD45 was only 15.2 nm long,[119] the fact that it is just larger than the actual separation of 13 nm means that this will induce near the maximal extent of exclusion that can be achieved through this physical process.

1.3.2   Phase-Separated Lipid Domains in Plasma Membrane

Roles of lipids in the structure of the immunological synapse have been proposed in addition to highly specific roles such as regulatory ligands that alter the conformation of receptors. In phospholipid bilayers, lipids may have acyl chain compositions that can undergo formation of liquid disordered (Ld) or liquid crystal (Lc) phases that display high lateral mobility or no lateral mobility, respectively. Addition of cholesterol to these systems converts the Ld phase into a liquid ordered (Lo) phase that displays intermediate lateral mobility.[127] There has been interest over the past 2 decades in how Lo phases in biological membrane may contribute to protein sorting and signaling in conjunction with protein-protein interactions.[128] Biochemical approaches to the fractionation of membranes based on relative resistance of Lo domains to detergents have been utilized with some success, but have also been criticized as having a risk of artifacts and caveats in correlation with native structures.[129] The scale and dynamics of these structures has made them a challenge for imaging, but homo-fluorescence resonance energy transfer by fluorescence anisotropy and dynamic and fixed super-resolution methods are now making inroads into physical characterization and determining the dimensions of Lo domains in biological membranes.[130–132] Many different antigen receptors, including the TCR, have been proposed to take advantage of Lo domains as signaling platforms. For examples, both Lck and LAT have lipid modifications that favor their entry into or nucleation of Lo domains. The transmembrane domain of CD45, in contrast, seems to favor its segregation from Lo domains, probably due to hydrophobic mismatch of the transmembrane domain with the deeper hydrophobic core of Lo domains.[131] Thus, in situations where CD45 cannot be excluded due to the size of its extracellular domain, it may be partly segregated based on its transmembrane domain under conditions where receptor cross-linking recruits Lo domains to the cluster.

1.3.3   Phase Separation in Membrane Proximal Signaling

The modular signaling components that are part of the cytoplasmic signaling complexes are built on multiple low-affinity interactions and assemble near the clustered receptors on a submicron length scale. One of the first signaling proteins for which phase-like behavior was demonstrated was WASP, a modular regulator of the Arp2/3 complex responsible for the expansion of branched F-actin networks.[122] While F-actin networks behave like solid gel phase structures, rather than liquid phases, the upstream regulators display liquid phase-like behavior. Recently, LAT-containing complexes have been shown to generate 2D phases that have lateral dimensions of micrometers but with depths of only a new 10's of nm.[133] These are very different from other cytoplasmic phase-like systems such as the nucleoli or p-granules, which are spherical.[121] This signaling phase-like layer near the membrane can then interface with cortical F-actin, which draws the LAT-mediated phases into elongated shapes.[133] Interestingly, these gel-liquid phase composites powerfully excluded CD45, seemingly on the basis of charge.[133] Thus, it is possible that the short-range exclusion of CD45 phosphatase domain from LAT phases could be a third mechanism to keep CD45 from snuffing out phosphotyrosine-based signaling complexes. Typically, phases are thought of as chemically accessible to soluble components, but in this example physical properties of the phase may allow another level of sorting of components out of or into local reaction centers.

1.3.4   Cytoskeletal Networks

Signaling events such as the trafficking of TCR microclusters in T cells during the formation and organization of the IS must be coordinated in time and space. These processes are known to heavily rely on active rearrangements of cytoskeletal networks at each stage.[15,27,134–142] The formation of actin-rich structures regulating membrane architecture of T cells are thought to be important during all three stages of cell activation including initial contact formation, IS formation, and contraction.[27,143]

The cytoskeleton of immune cells, like most animal cells, is composed of three classes of polymer networks: intermediate filaments, microtubules, and actin filaments (F-actin) constituting networks—of which in particular the latter two continuously undergo turnover of their protein components.[144,145] This holds notably for the actin cytoskeletal networks of immune cells that consist of the 3D cytoplasmic F-actin network and the cortical F-actin network, a submembranous shell that is the main determinant of cell shape and endows cells with their mechanical properties.[146,147] The cortex is a roughly isotropic polymeric network of semiflexible F-actin, which is cross-linked using specific F-actin-binding proteins and motor proteins generating stress within the network. Cells can respond quickly to external stimuli, both mechanical cues or biochemical signals using the repeated turnover of the filaments of cortical actin. As a consequence, the cortex plays a central role in division,[148,149] motility,[144,145] immune activation,[150] and many other biological processes internal to the cell.

In immune cells, the actin cytoskeleton forms four distinct structures: the actin cortex, contractile rings, lamellipodia, as well as lamella, and actin-rich protrusions.[147,151,152] These allow the cytoskeletal actin network, assisted by myosin-II proteins, to transduce chemical signals into mechanical force. In turn, the interplay between all of these factors facilitates reorganization and adjustment of F-actin networks in response to environmental cues.[152] The actin cortex is probably the most important actin structure, and it comprises polydisperse actin filaments undergoing constant turnover.[153,154] These actin dynamics involve either (i) the formin proteins, which associate with the fast-growing barbed end of long actin filaments resulting in their extension or (ii) the Arp2/3 complex, which is a nucleator of the branching of short actin filaments that is activated independently of formin by the Wiskott-Aldrich syndrome protein (WASp).[153] Through a dynamic interplay with myosin-II mini-filaments, the cortical network provides the cell with mechanical and structural integrity, and drives shape changes.[155] Contractile actin rings serve to pinch and separate daughter cells during cell division.[156] The lamellipodium, which is connected to the actin cortex by its lamellum, is a flat, highly dynamic structure comprised of mostly Arp2/3-nucleated actin filaments and a few structurally stabilizing, long formin-mediated filaments.[157]

We have recently characterized the nanoscale structure of the T-cell cortex with unprecedented detail and found that it is composed of two F-actin subpopulations, long formin-nucleated F-actin and short Arp2/3-nucleated F-actin with the ratio of populations and filament lengths changing on activation.[155] While the size of formin-nucleated filaments increased, the opposite effect was observed for the Arp2/3-mediated filaments. The observation that formin seems to stabilize IS formation is consistent with a previous analysis.[137,158,159] From a mechanical point of view, increasing the average length of larger formin-nucleated actin filaments likely produces a higher degree of cortical elasticity and therefore greater structural integrity and IS stability as well as a flatter and stiffer contact interface, a property that results in an efficient distribution of forces across the whole contact.[155,160] In contrast, shorter and dynamic Arp2/3-nucleated filaments, despite their higher abundance, usually contribute little to cortical elasticity.[155] However, they might contribute to a rapid reaction process allowing cells to respond for example, to TCR signaling by rapidly adjusting their turnover and length.[13,161] A relatively stiff cortex implies that T-cell activation and/or IS formation depends on the mechanical forces created by the actin cytoskeleton acting at the cell contact. Primary DCs form mechanosensitive podosomes at the contact periphery of the IS with T lymphocytes.[141,159] This supports the notion that T cells and DCs dynamically measure the stiffness of contact interfaces in order to adjust the underlying actin assembly dynamics, highlighting the requirement of precisely measuring mechanical forces at cell contacts (see e.g., [18,119,162–164]).

1.4 MICROVILLI/FILOPODIA

As a T cell approaches an APC or stimulatory substrate, the first contacts take place through F-actin-based projections, which can be ruffles or filopodia/microvilli. Nonpolarized lymphocytes isolated from blood or lymphoid tissues are studded with short projections that are ~0.4 μm long, 0.1 μm wide, and are present at a density of 3–4 μm^{-1}.[165] These are described as microvilli or filopodia based on their dimensions and F-actin dependence, as they collapse within 2 min of adding latrunculin A, a drug that sequesters F-actin monomers.[165,166] We will refer to these structures as filopodia as this description can be applied to longer structures at the leading edge of polarized cells or to the short structures on nonpolarized cells prior to contact with a stimulatory surface.[166] Recent superresolution microscopy studies have shown that on nonpolarized lymphocytes the TCR is concentrated on the tips of these projections.[167] This concentration of TCR at these sites perhaps explains earlier observations that the leading edge is the most sensitive part of a polarized T cell for the detection of p^{Ag}MHC or the action of stimulatory anti-CD3 antibodies.[168,169] In this setting, TCR colocalizes on these structures with L-selectin, which is well known to concentrate at the ends of projections (described as ruffles or microvilli) to facilitate its interaction with glycans on endothelial cells to establish rolling adhesion under flow conditions.[170] L-selectin is localized to projections at least in part through binding to ezrin-radixin-moesin (ERM) family cytoskeletal adapters.[171] The mechanism by which TCR localizes to these structures is not known, but vasodilator-stimulated phosphoprotein (VASP) proteins that localize to tips of the filopodia interact with the TCR.[138,172] This suggests that TCR and L-selection localization to projections may be regulated by different mechanisms in keeping with the different functional outcomes on engagement. TCR clustering on tips of projections may account for some of the nonuniform distribution of TCR observed by electron microscopy and total internal reflection fluorescence microscopy (TIRFM).[173,174] On the other hand, it is also possible that initial nonuniform distribution of TCR on flat membrane surfaces may nucleate the projections by recruiting proteins like VASP that can interact with F-actin nucleating factors. The formation of actin-based projections on T cells is independent of WASp and the growth of longer filopodia can be induced on T cells by overexpression of formins FRL2 and mDia2, but not mDia1.[165,166] However, the formins that are involved in the formation of steady-state projections in T cells remain to be determined. While the TCR and L-selectin are localized to projections on T cells, the integrins are localized to the flat surface between microvilli.[170] LFA-1 is also dependent upon formin-nucleated F-actin structures for its localization and function, but the specific formin involved is FHOD1,[18] which is not able to nucleate projections upon overexpression in T cells.[166] F-actin-based projections display dramatic dynamics on nano and microscales and have been proposed to execute systematic searches of surfaces contacted by T cells.[65,175] Whether the periodic extension and retraction of these protrusions generate the force needed to test TCR-p^{Ag}MHC catch bonds through application of ~10 pN force is not known. It is likely that these F-actin-based projections are the basis for the strong F-actin dependence of TCR microcluster formation induced by p^{Ag}MHC.[26,27]

Initial low-resolution views of early immunological synapse formation showed that LFA-1-ICAM-1-mediated adhesion appeared to be used as an anchor for cells to generate close contacts in which TCR-pMHC interactions were established through protrusive force.[10] Higher resolution views using TIRFM showed that TCR microclusters formed in the F-actin-rich regions of the interface with SLB containing ICAM-1 and p^{Ag}MHC.[27,46] Surprisingly, the formation and growth of TCR microclusters in response to surfaces with p^{Ag}MHC was not dependent on downstream signaling driven by SRC family kinases as it was resistant to inhibition by PP2.[27] The formation of TCR microclusters is F-actin dependent, but Arp2/3 independent based on resistance to CK666, an Arp2/3 complex inhibitor.[66] Even in the context of LFA-1-dependent adhesion, a "fractal" pattern of submicron protrusions was observed in cell-cell or cell-SLB interfaces with signaling independent stabilization of the protrusions resulting from p^{Ag}MHC-binding events.[65] The WASp- and Arp2/3-dependent generation of F-actin foci (also referred to as patches) at the TCR microclusters enhances downstream signaling associated with PLCγ activation and sustained calcium signaling.[66] Under conditions of low antigen density these structures develop a distinctive architecture in which each TCR microcluster is surrounded by its own microadhesion ring of LFA-1 and paxillin.[176] The higher the density of p^{Ag}MHC, the larger the growth of each microcluster. Once spreading is complete, F-actin polymerization that was initially involved in driving spreading converts into a centripetal F-actin flow that moves the TCR and integrin microslusters toward the center.[29,46,177] During this lateral transport, forces generated by F-actin polymerization and myosin-II-mediated contraction are likely exerted on both the integrin microclusters and the TCR microclusters, which may provide the necessary force to maintain high affinity conformation and catch bond activity, respectively.[158,178,179]

The F-actin foci associated with TCR microclusters have similarity to podosomes, which are thought to be force sensors that might assist cells in the decision processes regarding how to interact best with tissue surfaces of different mechanical properties.[180–182] Podosomes are also actin-rich, round structures at the vicinity of the basal plasma membrane. They are 0.5–2 μm in diameter and play an important role in cellular motility and invasion, and are typically found in cells that specialize in these features. From a structural point of view, podosomes have several characteristics: (1) Podosome formation can be induced in, for example, HeLa cells, where their appearance is not common, by overexpression of Src family kinases.[183] (2) Podosomes usually only appear at the cellular basal plane. (3) Podosomes have been shown to disappear completely in THP1 monocytes and do not undergo structural transitions following treatment by the Arp2/3-complex-inhibitor CK666.[184] (4). Myosin-II localizes to the arms and core of podosomes.[182] (5) Vinculin, a cytoskeletal protein strongly localizes to podosomes.[180]

In the case of lymphocytes, osteoclasts, and macrophages it has been shown that podosome formation has direct implications on their functioning.[159,180,182] This most likely follows from the fact that the organization of plasma membrane molecules, such as the receptors, is strongly influenced by the cortical actin network. The latter is, for example, the case for immune response, which is severely affected by the ability of the immune-relevant receptors to organize within the cell membrane. Their organization notably depends on the dynamics of the Arp2/3 complex and formins that control the ultra-structural properties of the cortical actin underlying the membrane. Formins may also contribute to the mechanical settings governing the formation and maintenance of actin patterns as the formins FHOD1 and INF2 have been recently demonstrated to control the de novo formation and contractility of podosomes.[185]

T lymphocytes do not form podosomes, but instead produce actin foci during the formation of the IS.[186,187] Kumari and colleagues recently demonstrated that they are polymerized de novo via a WASP-dependent mechanism.[66] Previously, it was proposed that similar TCR-associated F-actin foci were formed through a buildup of retrograde flowing F-actin moving over artificially immobilized TCR on chrome microbarriers in both Jurkat and primary T cells.[141] Foci enhance specific downstream TCR signaling steps, including PLCγ1 activation and calcium ion elevation, but are not required for TCR microcluster formation and other proximal signaling events such as ZAP-70 phosphorylation. Similar to podosomes, F-actin foci are depleted by WASP deficiency or CK666 treatment. In the case of both CD4 and CD8 primary T cells, the foci are robustly triggered following TCR ligation. In activated mouse T-cell blasts, antigen-dependent induction of foci was observed as well. In contrast to the primary T-cell systems, few foci are observed in Jurkat T cells. A signaling network linking TCR to WASP has been outlined in the Jurkat cells,[186] so it is likely this signaling pathway is intact. Interestingly, in Jurkat T cells, WASP is not required for the actin-polymerizing function related to calcium ion signaling (Silvin et al., 2001). Also, PLCγ1 activation[137] is not blocked by Arp2/3 silencing. Thus, it is possible that these cells utilize an alternative WASP-independent cytoskeletal pathway to support TCR-induced calcium ion elevation,[134] and therefore do not utilize foci in this way. Interestingly, Jurkat cells do form actin foci when formin-type F-actin nucleating factors are inhibited.[179] However, it was not determined how this impacted signaling. A detailed comparison of the differential organization and function of F-actin modalities comparing Jurkat cells and primary T cells is needed to comprehend the operation of compensatory cytoskeletal pathways associated with the assistance of TCR distal signaling and is likely important both at different developmental stages in the T-cell lineage and/ or in contributions to the deficiency of growth control in malignancy.

1.4.1 Rosette-Shaped Actin Network

The initial assessment of the F-actin network in synapse-forming T cells is based on (i) confocal microscopy of Jurkat T-cells expressing GFP-actin that revealed an expanding F-actin ring, (ii) edge-tracking algorithms of cells on stimulatory SLB that revealed lateral waves of extension, and (iii) retraction and speckle microscopy that revealed a coarse view of the underlying F-actin dynamics.[13,15,28,188] Lattice light sheet (LLS) imaging has also revealed significant F-actin dynamics outside the interface, which also needs to be considered in a full model for T-cell cytoskeletal contributions to activation.[143] Important details of the involvement of the actin cytoskeleton in T-cell activation remain unclear. (I) Whereas the lamellipodial actin flow and the localization of myosin-II motors at the basal plane of the lamellipodium have been described in detail,[13,134,158,179,189,190] their global (3D) organization across the whole cell remained largely unknown. (ii) The nanoscale organization of actin networks including meshwork sizes, F-actin turnover, and lengths of actin at each stage of T-cell activation remained uncharacterized. (iii) Transportation networks beneath the IS facilitating microcluster organization have so far not been reported in T cells, although these networks are generally believed to be connected to molecular transport.[191] Combining a range of advanced fluorescence microscopy tools including extended total internal reflection fluorescence-structured illumination microscopy, super-resolution stimulated emission depletion (STED) and LLS microscopy on resting and surface-activated Jurkat T cells, our group now can show that, in the course of their activation, the actin cytoskeleton of T cells undergoes a series of macroscopic and microscopic transformations rivaling the complexity of those accompanying eukaryotic cell division. These transformations involve (i) a global reorganization across the whole cell including the formation of each of the four main actin structures (cortex, ring, lamellipod, and spikes), (ii) the occurrence of a distinct inward-growing ramifying transportation-network of F-actin below the IS, whose dynamics are correlated with TCR and LFA-1 rearrangements (Fig. 1.1C), and (iii) distinct changes in actin filament lengths and meshwork sizes, suggesting that a high degree of cytoskeletal plasticity allows T cells to form cellular contacts at different length- and time-scales, and creating a very flat and particularly stiff contact. These observations are consistent with an older finding that T cells impose a flat cell–cell interface on B-cell lines that initially present a convex surface to the T cell.[192]

The location of the network 150–300 nm above the microscope cover glass explains why this structure has not been seen in conventional TIRFM studies, which penetrates only 50–100 nm into the sample. Unfortunately, we could not provide direct evidence for the ramified actin network to function as a transportation network because the ligands were fixed in place on the substrates. Simultaneous observation of TCR microcluster transportation and the propelling actin turnover dynamics of the ramified actin network remain technically challenging because they require dual-color super-resolution microscopy with extended spatial and substantial temporal resolution at a spatial location of 300 nm above the glass surface, which is beyond the technical possibilities of current super-resolution microscopy. The STED microscopy images confirmed the sequence of changes in the lamellipodium (i.e., spreading, undulation, contraction), but in addition revealed nanoscopic details of actin structure and rearrangement. Specifically, the STED microscopy images revealed that the symmetric contact observed in LLSM unfolded into a torus-shaped interface with the symmetric boundary required for strand formation and thus for growth inwards into the ramified actin network and outwards into the lamellipodium. Notably, previous super-resolution microscopy images of actin structures in other cell lines struggled to visualize such details of cortical networks owing to their dense cortical meshes (10–15 nm in, e.g., of cervical HeLa and melanoma cells[193]). The actin meshwork was readily resolved in Jurkat T cells owing to the much larger meshwork diameter of 150–200 nm in the cytosol and at the contact. In line with the mesh sizes observed using STED, the turnover rates and filament lengths of the cortical actin were fivefold larger in T cells than in non-lymphocytes ([154,155]). In fact, the authors found that T cells reorganize their nanoscale structures of the cortical actin network in response to antigen stimulation independent of the presence of a surface, for example, an APC. T cells suspended in a hydrogel away from any surface showed the same changes of the same magnitude in their F-actin lengths and turnover dynamics when activated with soluble antigens, suggesting that nanoscale changes of the actin cytoskeleton of T cells are independent of APCs, but are a result of specific activation with antigens.

The formation of the rosette-shaped F-actin network in 2D systems may be correlated with the observed deep F-actin lamellum observed in T-B conjugates.[194,195] F-actin regulatory elements play a key role in the control of a signaling pathway connecting protein kinase C-θ to NF-κB activation and the generation of active Notch intracellular domain. The recruitment of PKC-θ to engaged CD28 requires the F-actin uncapping regulator Rltpr.[196] Furthermore, PKC-θ then regulates the F-actin unbranching protein coronin-1 to regulate proteases that clear Notch.[197] Further analysis with 3D super-resolution methods may provide additional insight into how these F-actin rearrangements generate the appropriate forces to activate Notch in an apparently ligand-independent manner, which provides a key signal for T-cell proliferation.[117]

1.5 SYNAPTIC CLEFT FORMATION

One of the defining characteristics of the immunological synapse is directed secretion of effector molecules into an isolated space between the two cells.[1] This membrane traffic at the immunological synapse is thought to be focused not only by the F-actin cytoskeleton but also by the microtubule network at the microtubule organizing center (MTOC). Vesicular traffic is also critical for sustained T cell signaling and the generation of outside-out extracellular vesicles has recently been demonstrated to operate through at least three topological processes: exocytic vesicle fusion, endocytic vesicle formation, and extracellular vesicle budding, focused at the synaptic cleft.

1.5.1 Membrane Traffic to Maintain Signaling

All of the components needed to initiate T cell signaling are present in the plasma membrane as the T cells encounter stimulatory surfaces.[198] However, the dramatic rearrangement of the T-cell plasma membrane during immunological synapse formation includes the recruitment of new molecules, presumably to replace molecules that are spent in the first moments of signaling. As we will discuss below, individual TCR and many signaling components are consumed through ubiquitination and degradation, and new TCR and other components are needed to sustain signaling. The TCR is constitutively endocytosed and recycled back to the surface even in the absence of any pMHC ligands in cultured T cells.[199] Intracellular pools of vesicles bearing Lck and LAT are present in the steady state and maintained during T-cell activation.[200,201] Analysis of these compartments is complicated by their concentration near the MTOC, which translocates to the immunological synapse within minutes of initiating T-cell activation.[202–204] Nonetheless, a diversity of vesicles has been identified by careful analysis of confocal images and super-resolution microscopy data. Vesicles that fuse to the plasma membrane can be defined based on regulatory elements and fusogenic proteins that mark their cytoplasmic surface and target them to plasma membrane domains. A number of regulatory small G proteins are important for transport of these components: TCR with Rab8b (connects to Paxillin and Exocyst) > Rab3d (connects to IFTs and autophagy) > Rab4b (connects to TfR recycling); Lck with Rab11b (connects to receptor recycling), and LAT with Rab27a (a Rab controlling later exosome fusion to plasma membrane) > Rab35 (associated with filipodial extension).[205] Lck trafficking to the synapse was also associated with the integral membrane protein MAL, which has interactions with a number of other non-receptor tyrosine kinases.[205] The Rab3b-positive transport vesicles also have connections to the IFT20/57/88 complex defined recently by Baldari's laboratory as being critical for TCR recycling to sustain signaling.[206] In addition, Baldari defined Rab5 and IFT20 and Rab8a and VAMP3 dependent TCR recycling pathways that are important for sustained signaling.[207,208] Furthermore, the Hivroz laboratory has also found that recruitment of the vesicular pool of LAT to the immunological synapse required VAMP7.[209] The role of IFTs in TCR trafficking aligns with a model proposed by Griffiths that the immunological synapse acts as a provisional primary cilium during T-cell activation, which can also recruit signaling pathways such as Hedgehog to contribute to control of T-cell responses.[210] Finally, it has been proposed that vesicular pools of LAT may contribute to signaling through docking of the vesicles to signaling complexes without fusion.[211,212] When combined with protein phase-like behavior of LAT and its associated adapters, the docking of LAT-positive vesicles could generate 3D phase separated domains incorporating vesicles and F-actin to amplify signals, but this remains to be proven. This is clearly a very complex network of interactions, but the knowledge of functional markers for relevant compartments provides tools to appreciate further their functional importance.

1.5.2 Extracellular Vesicles to Terminate Signaling and Relay Messages

Signaling by individual TCRs is terminated after a couple of minutes in a process that requires the action of ubiquitin ligases.[213] The classical view of this process is that ubiquitinated TCR complexes are internalized and degraded in lysosomes[214]; however, loss of TCR from cells can also take place through the release of extracellular vesicles generated by the same endosomal sorting complexes required for the transport (ESCRT) system employed for protein sorting in lysosomal degradation. We found that TCR can be actively eliminated from T cells by ESCRT-dependent budding of vesicles directly into the synaptic cleft, while the TCR are still engaging $p^{Ag}MHC$[215] (Fig. 1.2). This process takes place in parallel with a trans-endocytosis mechanism in which TCR extract pMHC from the APC surface by a dynamin-dependent mechanism (Fig. 1.2). Eventually, TCR endocytosis will lead to the formation of exosomes, which can either be released into the synapse by exocytosis (again providing TCR+ vesicles to the APC).[216] We refer to vesicles that are directly budding into the plasma membrane without separation of TCR from pMHC as synaptic ectosomes to distinguish these from other types of exosomes that are generated in endosomal compartments and can be released into synapses or nondirectionally into the local tissue environment. Exosomes containing TCR are generated in a manner dependent upon the ESCRT-0 protein HRS,[216] suggesting a role for clathrin in the sorting mechanism in addition to ubiquitin.[217] Synaptic ectosomes released directly into the synaptic cleft do not require HRS, but do require ubiquitin recognition by tumor susceptibility gene-101.[218] Exosomes released in a Rab27a/b-independent manner has been observed as an effector mechanism for regulatory T cells based on the delivery by the exosomes of suppressive miRNAs to effector T cells.[219] We have found that the synaptic cleft contains multiple vesicle populations and have proposed that these may serve different roles in T-APC communication.[220] CD40L transfer from T cells to B cells has

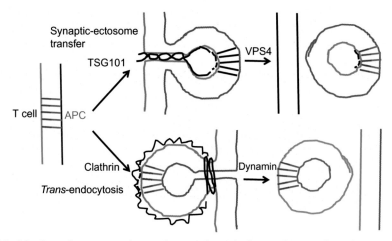

FIG. 1.2 Synaptic ectosome release and trans-endocytosis. See text for more discussion. The red lines represent TCR, whereas the blue lines represent pMHC. VPS4 is an ATPase that is involved in resolution of the bud neck in ESCRT-mediated vesicle budding. Dynamin is an ATPase involved in resolution of bud neck during endocytosis. Based on Choudhuri et al.,[215] both processes take place in T–B immunological synapse in vitro.

been observed in vitro and it was speculated that this takes place through synaptic extracellular vesicle transfer of some type.[221,222] Recently, we have found that dopamine-induced ICOSL on B cells induces increased CD40L accumulation in model immunological synapses formed on SLB with ICAM-1, anti-CD3, ICOSL, and CD40.[100] The form(s) of CD40L that is(are) relevant to T cell help requires further investigation. The cargo of extracellular vesicles includes miRNAs[216] and, by analogy to viral particles, may also contain metabolites that can convey information from cell to cell.[223]

1.5.3   Directed Release of Effector Molecules Through Exocytosis

In addition to the delivery of signaling molecules to maintain signaling, exocytic vesicle fusion also delivers critical effector molecules to the immunological synapse. Classic examples are the delivery of cytokines[6,224] and cytolytic molecules via directed secretion.[225] An interesting aspect of this is that cytolytic granules, which are a type of secretory lysosome,[226] are paired with endocytic vesicles[227] as a step in facilitating release; the endocytic vesicles can be TCR positive which may act as an additional safety mechanism to ensure that cytotoxic T cells deliver their cargo to antigen-positive cells.[228] In fact, an early proposal suggested that TCR-positive exosomes could be literally combined with cytotoxic cargo to ensure specificity.[229,230] More generally, the endosomes appear to provide priming factors[227,231] and utilize components, including VAMP8, which were discussed above in the context of sustained signaling.[232]

Application of mechanical force by cytotoxic T cells on target cells facilitates incorporation of perforin into the plasma membrane in a membrane tension-dependent manner.[162] This is a clear example of how mechanical force, generated by the ramified F-actin network, is part of the effector mechanisms utilized by T cells. There is still much to learn by applying even a more refined force measurement to T cells.[164,233]

1.6 CONCLUSIONS

The immunological synapse concept has evolved from early notions based on parallels in Ca^{2+} signaling and adhesion,[234] through early advances in digital fluorescent microscopy[2,10,27] and new features continue to be revealed with increasing spatial and temporal resolution.[65,233,235] There will continue to be fertile interplay between classical crystal structures, new methods such as cryo-electron microscopy and the suite of super-resolution microscopy methods in new discoveries regarding immunological synapses and kinapses.

ACKNOWLEDGMENTS

We thank our groups for stimulating data and discussions. MLD was supported by Wellcome Trust and Kennedy Trust for Rheumatology Research (PRF 100262Z/12/Z).

REFERENCES

1. Dustin ML, Colman DR. Neural and immunological synaptic relations. *Science* 2002;**298**:785–9.
2. Monks CR, Freiberg BA, Kupfer H, Sciaky N, Kupfer A. Three-dimensional segregation of supramolecular activation clusters in T cells. *Nature* 1998;**395**:82–6.
3. Stoll S, Delon J, Brotz TM, Germain RN. Dynamic imaging of T cell-dendritic cell interactions in lymph nodes. *Science* 2002;**296**:1873–6.
4. Davis DM, Dustin ML. What is the importance of the immunological synapse? *Trends Immunol* 2004;**25**:323–7.
5. Goodridge HS, Reyes CN, Becker CA, Katsumoto TR, Ma J, Wolf AJ, Bose N, Chan AS, Magee AS, Danielson ME, et al. Activation of the innate immune receptor Dectin-1 upon formation of a 'phagocytic synapse'. *Nature* 2011;**472**:471–5.
6. Huse M, Lillemeier BF, Kuhns MS, Chen DS, Davis MM. T cells use two directionally distinct pathways for cytokine secretion. *Nat Immunol* 2006;**7**:247–55.
7. Stinchcombe JC, Bossi G, Booth S, Griffiths GM. The immunological synapse of CTL contains a secretory domain and membrane bridges. *Immunity* 2001;**15**:751–61.
8. Carroll-Portillo A, Spendier K, Pfeiffer J, Griffiths G, Li H, Lidke KA, Oliver JM, Lidke DS, Thomas JL, Wilson BS, Timlin JA. Formation of a mast cell synapse: Fc epsilon RI membrane dynamics upon binding mobile or immobilized ligands on surfaces. *J Immunol* 2010;**184**:1328–38.
9. Davis DM, Chiu I, Fassett M, Cohen GB, Mandelboim O, Strominger JL. The human natural killer cell immune synapse. *Proc Natl Acad Sci U S A* 1999;**96**:15062–7.
10. Grakoui A, Bromley SK, Sumen C, Davis MM, Shaw AS, Allen PM, Dustin ML. The immunological synapse: a molecular machine controlling T cell activation. *Science* 1999;**285**:221–7.

11. Dushek O, Goyette J, van der Merwe PA. Non-catalytic tyrosine-phosphorylated receptors. *Immunol Rev* 2012;**250**:258–76.

12. Davis MM, Bjorkman PJ. T-cell antigen receptor genes and T-cell recognition. *Nature* 1988;**334**:395–402.

13. Sims TN, Soos TJ, Xenias HS, Dubin-Thaler B, Hofman JM, Waite JC, Cameron TO, Thomas VK, Varma R, Wiggins CH, et al. Opposing effects of PKCtheta and WASp on symmetry breaking and relocation of the immunological synapse. *Cell* 2007;**129**:773–85.

14. Freiberg BA, Kupfer H, Maslanik W, Delli J, Kappler J, Zaller DM, Kupfer A. Staging and resetting T cell activation in SMACs. *Nat Immunol* 2002;**3**:911–7.

15. Bunnell SC, Kapoor V, Trible RP, Zhang W, Samelson LE. Dynamic actin polymerization drives T cell receptor-induced spreading: a role for the signal transduction adaptor LAT. *Immunity* 2001;**14**:315–29.

16. Nguyen K, Sylvain NR, Bunnell SC. T cell costimulation via the integrin VLA-4 inhibits the actin-dependent centralization of signaling microclusters containing the adaptor SLP-76. *Immunity* 2008;**28**:810–21.

17. Husson J, Chemin K, Bohineust A, Hivroz C, Henry N. Force generation upon T cell receptor engagement. *PLoS One* 2011;**6**:e19680.

18. Tabdanov E, Gondarenko S, Kumari S, Liapis A, Dustin ML, Sheetz MP, Kam LC, Iskratsch T. Micropatterning of TCR and LFA-1 ligands reveals complementary effects on cytoskeleton mechanics in T cells. *Integr Biol (Camb)* 2015;**7**:1272–84.

19. Azar GA, Lemaitre F, Robey EA, Bousso P. Subcellular dynamics of T cell immunological synapses and kinapses in lymph nodes. *Proc Natl Acad Sci U S A* 2010;**107**:3675–80.

20. Dustin ML. Cell adhesion molecules and actin cytoskeleton at immune synapses and kinapses. *Curr Opin Cell Biol* 2007;**19**:529–33.

21. Dustin ML. Hunter to gatherer and back: immunological synapses and kinapses as variations on the theme of amoeboid locomotion. *Annu Rev Cell Dev Biol* 2008;**24**:577–96.

22. Dustin ML. T-cell activation through immunological synapses and kinapses. *Immunol Rev* 2008;**221**:77–89.

23. Halle S, Keyser KA, Stahl FR, Busche A, Marquardt A, Zheng X, Galla M, Heissmeyer V, Heller K, Boelter J, et al. In vivo killing capacity of cytotoxic T cells is limited and involves dynamic interactions and T cell cooperativity. *Immunity* 2016;**44**:233–45.

24. Brossard C, Feuillet V, Schmitt A, Randriamampita C, Romao M, Raposo G, Trautmann A. Multifocal structure of the T cell—dendritic cell synapse. *Eur J Immunol* 2005;**35**: 1741–53.

25. Tseng SY, Waite JC, Liu M, Vardhana S, Dustin ML. T cell-dendritic cell immunological synapses contain TCR-dependent CD28-CD80 clusters that recruit protein kinase Ctheta. *J Immunol* 2008;**181**:4852–63.

26. Bunnell SC, Hong DI, Kardon JR, Yamazaki T, McGlade CJ, Barr VA, Samelson LE. T cell receptor ligation induces the formation of dynamically regulated signaling assemblies. *J Cell Biol* 2002;**158**:1263–75.

27. Campi G, Varma R, Dustin ML. Actin and agonist MHC-peptide complex-dependent T cell receptor microclusters as scaffolds for signaling. *J Exp Med* 2005;**202**:1031–6.

28. Kaizuka Y, Douglass AD, Varma R, Dustin ML, Vale RD. Mechanisms for segregating T cell receptor and adhesion molecules during immunological synapse formation in Jurkat T cells. *Proc Natl Acad Sci U S A* 2007;**104**:20296–301.

29. Yokosuka T, Sakata-Sogawa K, Kobayashi W, Hiroshima M, Hashimoto-Tane A, Tokunaga M, Dustin ML, Saito T. Newly generated T cell receptor microclusters initiate and sustain T cell activation by recruitment of Zap70 and SLP-76. *Nat Immunol* 2005;**6**:1253–62.

30. Hashimoto-Tane A, Yokosuka T, Sakata-Sogawa K, Sakuma M, Ishihara C, Tokunaga M, Saito T. Dynein-driven transport of T cell receptor microclusters regulates immune synapse formation and T cell activation. *Immunity* 2011;**34**:919–31.

31. Kuhn JR, Poenie M. Dynamic polarization of the microtubule cytoskeleton during CTL-mediated killing. *Immunity* 2002;**16**:111–21.

32. Yi J, Wu X, Chung AH, Chen JK, Kapoor TM, Hammer JA. Centrosome repositioning in T cells is biphasic and driven by microtubule end-on capture-shrinkage. *J Cell Biol* 2013;**202**:779–92.

33. Sandstrom A, Peigne CM, Leger A, Crooks JE, Konczak F, Gesnel MC, Breathnach R, Bonneville M, Scotet E, Adams EJ. The intracellular B30.2 domain of butyrophilin 3A1 binds phosphoantigens to mediate activation of human Vgamma9Vdelta2 T cells. *Immunity* 2014;**40**:490–500.

34. Mattner J, Debord KL, Ismail N, Goff RD, Cantu 3rd C, Zhou D, Saint-Mezard P, Wang V, Gao Y, Yin N, et al. Exogenous and endogenous glycolipid antigens activate NKT cells during microbial infections. *Nature* 2005;**434**:525–9.

35. Corbett AJ, Eckle SB, Birkinshaw RW, Liu L, Patel O, Mahony J, Chen Z, Reantragoon R, Meehan B, Cao H, et al. T-cell activation by transitory neo-antigens derived from distinct microbial pathways. *Nature* 2014;**509**:361–5.

36. Zehn D, Bevan MJ. T cells with low avidity for a tissue-restricted antigen routinely evade central and peripheral tolerance and cause autoimmunity. *Immunity* 2006;**25**:261–70.

37. Liu B, Zhong S, Malecek K, Johnson LA, Rosenberg SA, Zhu C, Krogsgaard M. 2D TCR-pMHC-CD8 kinetics determines T-cell responses in a self-antigen-specific TCR system. *Eur J Immunol* 2014;**44**:239–50.

38. Morris GP, Allen PM. How the TCR balances sensitivity and specificity for the recognition of self and pathogens. *Nat Immunol* 2012;**13**:121–8.

39. Hogquist KA, Jameson SC. The self-obsession of T cells: how TCR signaling thresholds affect fate 'decisions' and effector function. *Nat Immunol* 2014;**15**:815–23.

40. Legoux FP, Lim JB, Cauley AW, Dikiy S, Ertelt J, Mariani TJ, Sparwasser T, Way SS, Moon JJ. CD4+ T cell tolerance to tissue-restricted self antigens is mediated by antigen-specific regulatory T cells rather than deletion. *Immunity* 2015;**43**:896–908.

41. Su LF, Kidd BA, Han A, Kotzin JJ, Davis MM. Virus-specific CD4(+) memory-phenotype T cells are abundant in unexposed adults. *Immunity* 2013;**38**:373–83.

42. Yu W, Jiang N, Ebert PJ, Kidd BA, Muller S, Lund PJ, Juang J, Adachi K, Tse T, Birnbaum ME, et al. Clonal deletion prunes but does not eliminate self-specific alphabeta CD8(+) T lymphocytes. *Immunity* 2015;**42**:929–41.

43. Qi S, Krogsgaard M, Davis MM, Chakraborty AK. Molecular flexibility can influence the stimulatory ability of receptor-ligand interactions at cell-cell junctions. *Proc Natl Acad Sci U S A* 2006;**103**:4416–21.

44. Garcia KC, Degano M, Stanfield RL, Brunmark A, Jackson MR, Peterson PA, Teyton L, Wilson IA. An alphabeta T cell receptor structure at 2.5 A and its orientation in the TCR-MHC complex. *Science* 1996;**274**:209–19.

45. Huppa JB, Axmann M, Mortelmaier MA, Lillemeier BF, Newell EW, Brameshuber M, Klein LO, Schutz GJ, Davis MM. TCR-peptide-MHC interactions in situ show accelerated kinetics and increased affinity. *Nature* 2010;**463**:963–7.

46. Varma R, Campi G, Yokosuka T, Saito T, Dustin ML. T cell receptor-proximal signals are sustained in peripheral microclusters and terminated in the central supramolecular activation cluster. *Immunity* 2006;**25**:117–27.

47. Dembo M, Torney DC, Saxman K, Hammer D. The reaction-limited kinetics of membrane-to-surface adhesion and detachment. *Proc R Soc Lond Ser B* 1988;**234**:55–83.

48. Das DK, Feng Y, Mallis RJ, Li X, Keskin DB, Hussey RE, Brady SK, Wang JH, Wagner G, Reinherz EL, Lang MJ. Force-dependent transition in the T-cell receptor beta-subunit allosterically regulates peptide discrimination and pMHC bond lifetime. *Proc Natl Acad Sci U S A* 2015;**112**:1517–22.

49. Liu B, Chen W, Evavold BD, Zhu C. Accumulation of dynamic catch bonds between TCR and agonist peptide-MHC triggers T cell signaling. *Cell* 2014;**157**:357–68.

50. Das DK, Mallis RJ, Duke-Cohan JS, Hussey RE, Tetteh PW, Hilton M, Wagner G, Lang MJ, Reinherz EL. Pre-T cell receptors (pre-TCRs) leverage Vbeta complementarity determining regions (CDRs) and hydrophobic patch in mechanosensing thymic self-ligands. *J Biol Chem* 2016;**291**:25292–305.

51. Kim ST, Takeuchi K, Sun ZY, Touma M, Castro CE, Fahmy A, Lang MJ, Wagner G, Reinherz EL. The alphabeta T cell receptor is an anisotropic mechanosensor. *J Biol Chem* 2009;**284**:31028–37.

52. Li YC, Chen BM, Wu PC, Cheng TL, Kao LS, Tao MH, Lieber A, Roffler SR. Cutting edge: mechanical forces acting on T cells immobilized via the TCR complex can trigger TCR signaling. *J Immunol* 2010;**184**:5959–63.

53. Bachmann MF, Barner M, Kopf M. CD2 sets quantitative thresholds in T cell activation. *J Exp Med* 1999;**190**:1383–92.

54. Irvine DJ, Purbhoo MA, Krogsgaard M, Davis MM. Direct observation of ligand recognition by T cells. *Nature* 2002;**419**:845–9.

55. Springer TA, Dustin ML. Integrin inside-out signaling and the immunological synapse. *Curr Opin Cell Biol* 2011;**24**:107–15.

56. Kinashi T, Aker M, Sokolovsky-Eisenberg M, Grabovsky V, Tanaka C, Shamri R, Feigelson S, Etzioni A, Alon R. LAD-III, a leukocyte adhesion deficiency syndrome associated with defective Rap1 activation and impaired stabilization of integrin bonds. *Blood* 2004;**103**:1033–6.

57. Kishimoto TK, Hollander N, Roberts TM, Anderson DC, Springer TA. Heterogeneous mutations in the beta subunit common to the LFA-1, Mac-1, and p150,95 glycoproteins cause leukocyte adhesion deficiency. *Cell* 1987;**50**:193–202.

58. Guttman-Yassky E, Vugmeyster Y, Lowes MA, Chamian F, Kikuchi T, Kagen M, Gilleaudeau P, Lee E, Hunte B, Howell K, et al. Blockade of CD11a by efalizumab in psoriasis patients induces a unique state of T-cell hyporesponsiveness. *J Invest Dermatol* 2008;**128**:1182–91.

59. Major EO. Progressive multifocal leukoencephalopathy in patients on immunomodulatory therapies. *Annu Rev Med* 2009;**61**:35–47.

60. Shimaoka M, Xiao T, Liu JH, Yang Y, Dong Y, Jun CD, McCormack A, Zhang R, Joachimiak A, Takagi J, et al. Structures of the alpha L I domain and its complex with ICAM-1 reveal a shape-shifting pathway for integrin regulation. *Cell* 2003;**112**:99–111.

61. Nishida N, Xie C, Shimaoka M, Cheng Y, Walz T, Springer TA. Activation of leukocyte beta2 integrins by conversion from bent to extended conformations. *Immunity* 2006;**25**:583–94.

62. Staunton DE, Marlin SD, Stratowa C, Dustin ML, Springer TA. Primary structure of ICAM-1 demonstrates interaction between members of the immunoglobulin and integrin supergene families. *Cell* 1988;**52**:925–33.

63. Zhu J, Luo BH, Xiao T, Zhang C, Nishida N, Springer TA. Structure of a complete integrin ectodomain in a physiologic resting state and activation and deactivation by applied forces. *Mol Cell* 2008;**32**:849–61.

64. Staunton DE, Dustin ML, Springer TA. Functional cloning of ICAM-2, a cell adhesion ligand for LFA-1 homologous to ICAM-1. *Nature* 1989;**339**:61–4.

65. Cai E, Marchuk K, Beemiller P, Beppler C, Rubashkin MG, Weaver VM, Gerard A, Liu TL, Chen BC, Betzig E, et al. Visualizing dynamic microvillar search and stabilization during ligand detection by T cells. *Science* 2017;**356**. eaal3118.

66. Kumari S, Depoil D, Martinelli R, Judokusumo E, Carmona G, Gertler FB, Kam LC, Carman CV, Burkhardt JK, Irvine DJ, Dustin ML. Actin foci facilitate activation of the phospholipase C-gamma in primary T lymphocytes via the WASP pathway. *elife* 2015;**4**: e04953.

67. Dustin ML, Sanders ME, Shaw S, Springer TA. Purified lymphocyte function-associated antigen 3 binds to CD2 and mediates T lymphocyte adhesion. *J Exp Med* 1987;**165**:677–92.

68. van der Merwe PA, Barclay AN, Mason DW, Davies EA, Morgan BP, Tone M, Krishnam AK, Ianelli C, Davis SJ. Human cell-adhesion molecule CD2 binds CD58 (LFA-3) with a very low affinity and an extremely fast dissociation rate but does not bind CD48 or CD59. *Biochemistry* 1994;**33**:10149–60.

69. Wang JH, Smolyar A, Tan K, Liu JH, Kim M, Sun ZY, Wagner G, Reinherz EL. Structure of a heterophilic adhesion complex between the human CD2 and CD58 (LFA-3) counterreceptors. *Cell* 1999;**97**:791–803.

70. Brown MH, Boles K, van der Merwe PA, Kumar V, Mathew PA, Barclay AN. 2B4, the natural killer and T cell immunoglobulin superfamily surface protein, is a ligand for CD48. *J Exp Med* 1998;**188**:2083–90.

71. Dustin ML, Golan DE, Zhu DM, Miller JM, Meier W, Davies EA, van der Merwe PA. Low affinity interaction of human or rat T cell adhesion molecule CD2 with its ligand aligns adhering membranes to achieve high physiological affinity. *J Biol Chem* 1997;**272**:30889–98.

72. Green JM, Karpitskiy V, Kimzey SL, Shaw AS. Coordinate regulation of T cell activation by CD2 and CD28. *J Immunol* 2000;**164**:3591–5.

73. Choudhuri K, Wiseman D, Brown MH, Gould K, van der Merwe PA. T-cell receptor triggering is critically dependent on the dimensions of its peptide-MHC ligand. *Nature* 2005;**436**:578–82.

74. Milstein O, Tseng SY, Starr T, Llodra J, Nans A, Liu M, Wild MK, van der Merwe PA, Stokes DL, Reisner Y, Dustin ML. Nanoscale increases in CD2-CD48-mediated intermembrane spacing decrease adhesion and reorganize the immunological synapse. *J Biol Chem* 2008;**283**:34414–22.

75. Bell GI. Models for the specific adhesion of cells to cells. *Science* 1978;**200**:618–27.

76. Dustin ML, Ferguson LM, Chan PY, Springer TA, Golan DE. Visualization of CD2 interaction with LFA-3 and determination of the two-dimensional dissociation constant for adhesion receptors in a contact area. *J Cell Biol* 1996;**132**:465–74.

77. Dustin ML, Starr T, Coombs D, Majeau GR, Meier W, Hochman PS, Douglass A, Vale R, Goldstein B, Whitty A. Quantification and modeling of tripartite CD2-, CD58FC chimera (Alefacept)-, and CD16-mediated cell adhesion. *J Biol Chem* 2007;**282**:34748–57.

78. Shaw AS, Dustin ML. Making the T cell receptor go the distance: a topological view of T cell activation. *Immunity* 1997;**6**:361–9.

79. Wild MK, Cambiaggi A, Brown MH, Davies EA, Ohno H, Saito T, van der Merwe PA. Dependence of T cell antigen recognition on the dimensions of an accessory receptor-ligand complex. *J Exp Med* 1999;**190**:31–41.

80. McKinney EF, Lee JC, Jayne DR, Lyons PA, Smith KG. T-cell exhaustion, co-stimulation and clinical outcome in autoimmunity and infection. *Nature* 2015;**523**:612–616.

81. Dustin ML, Olszowy MW, Holdorf AD, Li J, Bromley S, Desai N, Widder P, Rosenberger F, van der Merwe PA, Allen PM, Shaw AS. A novel adapter protein orchestrates receptor patterning and cytoskeletal polarity in T cell contacts. *Cell* 1998;**94**:667–77.

82. Dustin ML, Olive D, Springer TA. Correlation of CD2 binding and functional properties of multimeric and monomeric lymphocyte function-associated antigen 3. *J Exp Med* 1989;**169**:503–17.

83. Kaizuka Y, Douglass AD, Vardhana S, Dustin ML, Vale RD. The coreceptor CD2 uses plasma membrane microdomains to transduce signals in T cells. *J Cell Biol* 2009;**185**:521–34.

84. Latour S, Roncagalli R, Chen R, Bakinowski M, Shi X, Schwartzberg PL, Davidson D, Veillette A. Binding of SAP SH2 domain to FynT SH3 domain reveals a novel mechanism of receptor signalling in immune regulation. *Nat Cell Biol* 2003;**5**:149–54.

85. Pachlopnik Schmid J, Canioni D, Moshous D, Touzot F, Mahlaoui N, Hauck F, Kanegane H, Lopez-Granados E, Mejstrikova E, Pellier I, et al. Clinical similarities and differences of patients with X-linked lymphoproliferative syndrome type 1 (XLP-1/SAP deficiency) versus type 2 (XLP-2/XIAP deficiency). *Blood* 2011;**117**:1522–9.

86. Li C, Iosef C, Jia CY, Han VK, Li SS. Dual functional roles for the X-linked lymphoproliferative syndrome gene product SAP/SH2D1A in signaling through the signaling lymphocyte activation molecule (SLAM) family of immune receptors. *J Biol Chem* 2003;**278**:3852–9.

87. Pasquier B, Yin L, Fondaneche MC, Relouzat F, Bloch-Queyrat C, Lambert N, Fischer A, de Saint-Basile G, Latour S. Defective NKT cell development in mice and humans lacking the adapter SAP, the X-linked lymphoproliferative syndrome gene product. *J Exp Med* 2005;**201**:695–701.

88. Yan Q, Malashkevich VN, Fedorov A, Fedorov E, Cao E, Lary JW, Cole JL, Nathenson SG, Almo SC. Structure of CD84 provides insight into SLAM family function. *Proc Natl Acad Sci U S A* 2007;**104**:10583–8.

89. Zhao F, Cannons JL, Dutta M, Griffiths GM, Schwartzberg PL. Positive and negative signaling through SLAM receptors regulate synapse organization and thresholds of cytolysis. *Immunity* 2012;**36**:1003–16.

90. Riley JL, June CH. The CD28 family: a T-cell rheostat for therapeutic control of T-cell activation. *Blood* 2005;**105**:13–21.

91. Bromley SK, Iaboni A, Davis SJ, Whitty A, Green JM, Shaw AS, Weiss A, Dustin ML. The immunological synapse and CD28-CD80 interactions. *Nat Immunol* 2001;**2**:1159–66.

92. Qureshi OS, Zheng Y, Nakamura K, Attridge K, Manzotti C, Schmidt EM, Baker J, Jeffery LE, Kaur S, Briggs Z, et al. Trans-endocytosis of CD80 and CD86: a molecular basis for the cell-extrinsic function of CTLA-4. *Science* 2011;**332**:600–3.

93. Hui E, Cheung J, Zhu J, Su X, Taylor MJ, Wallweber HA, Sasmal DK, Huang J, Kim JM, Mellman I, Vale RD. T cell costimulatory receptor CD28 is a primary target for PD-1-mediated inhibition. *Science* 2017;**355**:1428–1433.

94. Saha A, O'Connor RS, Thangavelu G, Lovitch SB, Dandamudi DB, Wilson CB, Vincent BG, Tkachev V, Pawlicki JM, Furlan SN, et al. Programmed death ligand-1 expression on donor T cells drives graft-versus-host disease lethality. *J Clin Invest* 2016;**126**:2642–60.

95. Kamphorst AO, Wieland A, Nasti T, Yang S, Zhang R, Barber DL, Konieczny BT, Daugherty CZ, Koenig L, Yu K, et al. Rescue of exhausted CD8 T cells by PD-1-targeted therapies is CD28-dependent. *Science* 2017;**355**:1423–7.

96. Larkin J, Chiarion-Sileni V, Gonzalez R, Grob JJ, Cowey CL, Lao CD, Schadendorf D, Dummer R, Smylie M, Rutkowski P, et al. Combined nivolumab and ipilimumab or monotherapy in untreated melanoma. *N Engl J Med* 2015;**373**:23–34.

97. Maue AC, Yager EJ, Swain SL, Woodland DL, Blackman MA, Haynes L. T-cell immunosenescence: lessons learned from mouse models of aging. *Trends Immunol* 2009;**30**:301–5.

98. Izawa K, Martin E, Soudais C, Bruneau J, Boutboul D, Rodriguez R, Lenoir C, Hislop AD, Besson C, Touzot F, et al. Inherited CD70 deficiency in humans reveals a critical role for the CD70-CD27 pathway in immunity to Epstein-Barr virus infection. *J Exp Med* 2017;**214**:73–89.

99. Liu D, Xu H, Shih C, Wan Z, Ma X, Ma W, Luo D, Qi H. T-B-cell entanglement and ICOSL-driven feed-forward regulation of germinal centre reaction. *Nature* 2015;**517**:214–8.

100. Papa I, Saliba D, Ponzoni M, Bustamante S, Canete PF, Gonzalez-Figueroa P, McNamara HA, Valvo S, Grimbaldeston M, Sweet RA, et al. TFH-derived dopamine accelerates productive synapses in germinal centres. *Nature* 2017;**547**:318–23.

101. Quezada SA, Jarvinen LZ, Lind EF, Noelle RJ. CD40/CD154 interactions at the interface of tolerance and immunity. *Annu Rev Immunol* 2004;**22**:307–28.

102. Nocentini G, Riccardi C. GITR: a multifaceted regulator of immunity belonging to the tumor necrosis factor receptor superfamily. *Eur J Immunol* 2005;**35**:1016–22.

103. Byun M, Ma CS, Akcay A, Pedergnana V, Palendira U, Myoung J, Avery DT, Liu Y, Abhyankar A, Lorenzo L, et al. Inherited human OX40 deficiency underlying classic Kaposi sarcoma of childhood. *J Exp Med* 2013;**210**:1743–59.

104. Porter DL, Levine BL, Kalos M, Bagg A, June CH. Chimeric antigen receptor-modified T cells in chronic lymphoid leukemia. *N Engl J Med* 2011;**365**:725–33.

105. Samanta D, Ramagopal UA, Rubinstein R, Vigdorovich V, Nathenson SG, Almo SC. Structure of Nectin-2 reveals determinants of homophilic and heterophilic interactions that control cell-cell adhesion. *Proc Natl Acad Sci U S A* 2012;**109**:14836–40.

106. Takeuchi A, Badr Mel S, Miyauchi K, Ishihara C, Onishi R, Guo Z, Sasaki Y, Ike H, Takumi A, Tsuji NM, et al. CRTAM determines the CD4+ cytotoxic T lymphocyte lineage. *J Exp Med* 2016;**213**:123–38.

107. Rosen SD. Ligands for L-selectin: homing, inflammation, and beyond. *Annu Rev Immunol* 2004;**22**:129–56.

108. Sarafova SD, Erman B, Yu Q, Van Laethem F, Guinter T, Sharrow SO, Feigenbaum L, Wildt KF, Ellmeier W, Singer A. Modulation of coreceptor transcription during positive selection dictates lineage fate independently of TCR/coreceptor specificity. *Immunity* 2005;**23**:75–87.

109. Jonsson P, Southcombe JH, Santos AM, Huo J, Fernandes RA, McColl J, Lever M, Evans EJ, Hudson A, Chang VT, et al. Remarkably low affinity of CD4/peptide-major histocompatibility complex class II protein interactions. *Proc Natl Acad Sci U S A* 2016;**113**:5682–5687.

110. Stepanek O, Prabhakar AS, Osswald C, King CG, Bulek A, Naeher D, Beaufils-Hugot M, Abanto ML, Galati V, Hausmann B, et al. Coreceptor scanning by the T cell receptor provides a mechanism for T cell tolerance. *Cell* 2014;**159**:333–45.

111. Sicheri F, Moarefi I, Kuriyan J. Crystal structure of the Src family tyrosine kinase Hck. *Nature* 1997;**385**:602–9.

112. Bergman M, Mustelin T, Oetken C, Partanen J, Flint NA, Amrein KE, Autero M, Burn P, Alitalo K. The human p50csk tyrosine kinase phosphorylates p56lck at Tyr-505 and down regulates its catalytic activity. *EMBO J* 1992;**11**:2919–24.

113. Kawabuchi M, Satomi Y, Takao T, Shimonishi Y, Nada S, Nagai K, Tarakhovsky A, Okada M. Transmembrane phosphoprotein Cbp regulates the activities of Src-family tyrosine kinases. *Nature* 2000;**404**:999–1003.

114. Mustelin T, Altman A. Dephosphorylation and activation of the T cell tyrosine kinase pp56lck by the leukocyte common antigen (CD45). *Oncogene* 1990;**5**:809–13.

115. Shah NH, Wang Q, Yan Q, Karandur D, Kadlecek TA, Fallahee IR, Russ WP, Ranganathan R, Weiss A, Kuriyan J. An electrostatic selection mechanism controls sequential kinase signaling downstream of the T cell receptor. *elife* 2016;**5**: e20105.

116. Schaeffer EM, Yap GS, Lewis CM, Czar MJ, McVicar DW, Cheever AW, Sher A, Schwartzberg PL. Mutation of Tec family kinases alters T helper cell differentiation. *Nat Immunol* 2001;**2**:1183–8.

117. Guy CS, Vignali KM, Temirov J, Bettini ML, Overacre AE, Smeltzer M, Zhang H, Huppa JB, Tsai YH, Lobry C, et al. Distinct TCR signaling pathways drive proliferation and cytokine production in T cells. *Nat Immunol* 2013;**14**:262–70.
118. James JR, Vale RD. Biophysical mechanism of T-cell receptor triggering in a reconstituted system. *Nature* 2012;**487**:64–9.
119. Chang VT, Fernandes RA, Ganzinger KA, Lee SF, Siebold C, McColl J, Jonsson P, Palayret M, Harlos K, Coles CH, et al. Initiation of T cell signaling by CD45 segregation at 'close contacts'. *Nat Immunol* 2016;**17**:574–82.
120. Dustin ML, Choudhuri K. Signaling and polarized communication across the T cell immunological synapse. *Annu Rev Cell Dev Biol* 2016;**32**:303–325.
121. Brangwynne CP, Mitchison TJ, Hyman AA. Active liquid-like behavior of nucleoli determines their size and shape in Xenopus laevis oocytes. *Proc Natl Acad Sci U S A* 2011;**108**:4334–9.
122. Li P, Banjade S, Cheng HC, Kim S, Chen B, Guo L, Llaguno M, Hollingsworth JV, King DS, Banani SF, et al. Phase transitions in the assembly of multivalent signalling proteins. *Nature* 2012;**483**:336–40.
123. Clausen MP, Colin-York H, Schneider F, Eggeling C, Fritzsche M. Dissecting the actin cortex density and membrane-cortex distance in living cells by super-resolution microscopy. *J Phys D Appl Phys* 2017;**50**:064002.
124. Dustin ML. Adhesive bond dynamics in contacts between T lymphocytes and glass supported planar bilayers reconstituted with the immunoglobulin related adhesion molecule CD58. *J Biol Chem* 1997;**272**:15782–8.
125. Burroughs NJ, Kohler K, Miloserdov V, Dustin ML, van der Merwe PA, Davis DM. Boltzmann energy-based image analysis demonstrates that extracellular domain size differences explain protein segregation at immune synapses. *PLoS Comput Biol* 2011;**7**:e1002076.
126. Schmid EM, Bakalar MH, Choudhuri K, Weichsel J, Ann H, Geissler PL, Dustin ML, Fletcher DA. Size-dependent protein segregation at membrane interfaces. *Nat Phys* 2016;**12**:704–11.
127. Sezgin E, Levental I, Grzybek M, Schwarzmann G, Mueller V, Honigmann A, Belov VN, Eggeling C, Coskun U, Simons K, Schwille P. Partitioning, diffusion, and ligand binding of raft lipid analogs in model and cellular plasma membranes. *Biochim Biophys Acta* 2012;**1818**:1777–84.
128. Simons K, Ikonen E. Functional rafts in cell membranes. *Nature* 1997;**387**:569–72.
129. Brown DA, London E. Structure and function of sphingolipid- and cholesterol-rich membrane rafts. *J Biol Chem* 2000;**275**:17221–4.
130. Eggeling C, Ringemann C, Medda R, Schwarzmann G, Sandhoff K, Polyakova S, Belov VN, Hein B, von Middendorff C, Schonle A, Hell SW. Direct observation of the nanoscale dynamics of membrane lipids in a living cell. *Nature* 2009;**457**:1159–62.
131. Stone MB, Shelby SA, Nunez MF, Wisser K, Veatch SL. Protein sorting by lipid phase-like domains supports emergent signaling function in B lymphocyte plasma membranes. *elife* 2017;**6**: e19891.
132. Varma R, Mayor S. GPI-anchored proteins are organized in submicron domains at the cell surface. *Nature* 1998;**394**:798–801.
133. Su X, Ditlev JA, Hui E, Xing W, Banjade S, Okrut J, King DS, Taunton J, Rosen MK, Vale RD. Phase separation of signaling molecules promotes T cell receptor signal transduction. *Science* 2016;**352**:595–9.
134. Babich A, Li S, O'Connor RS, Milone MC, Freedman BD, Burkhardt JK. F-actin polymerization and retrograde flow drive sustained PLCgamma1 signaling during T cell activation. *J Cell Biol* 2012;**197**:775–87.

135. Billadeau DD, Nolz JC, Gomez TS. Regulation of T-cell activation by the cytoskeleton. *Nat Rev Immunol* 2007;**7**:131–43.

136. Cannon JL, Burkhardt JK. The regulation of actin remodeling during T-cell-APC conjugate formation. *Immunol Rev* 2002;**186**:90–9.

137. Gomez TS, Kumar K, Medeiros RB, Shimizu Y, Leibson PJ, Billadeau DD. Formins regulate the actin-related protein 2/3 complex-independent polarization of the centrosome to the immunological synapse. *Immunity* 2007;**26**:177–90.

138. Krause M, Sechi AS, Konradt M, Monner D, Gertler FB, Wehland J. Fyn-binding protein (Fyb)/SLP-76-associated protein (SLAP), Ena/vasodilator-stimulated prosphoprotein (VASP) proteins and the Arp2/3 complex link T cell receptor (TCR) signaling to the actin cytoskeleton. *JCell Biol* 2000;**149**:181–94.

139. Reicher B, Barda-Saad M. Multiple pathways leading from the T-cell antigen receptor to the actin cytoskeleton network. *FEBS Lett* 2010;**584**:4858–64.

140. Schwartzberg PL. Formin the way. *Immunity* 2007;**26**:139–41.

141. Smoligovets AA, Smith AW, Wu H-J, Petit RS, Groves JT. Characterization of dynamic actin associations with T-cell receptor microclusters in primary T cells. *J Cell Sci* 2012;**125**:735–42.

142. Yu Y, Smoligovets AA, Groves JT. Modulation of T cell signaling by the actin cytoskeleton. *J Cell Sci* 2013;**126**:1049–58.

143. Ritter AT, Asano Y, Stinchcombe JC, Dieckmann NM, Chen BC, Gawden-Bone C, van Engelenburg S, Legant W, Gao L, Davidson MW, et al. Actin depletion initiates events leading to granule secretion at the immunological synapse. *Immunity* 2015;**42**:864–76.

144. Charras G. A short history of blebbing. *J Microsc* 2008;**231**:466–78.

145. Pollard TD, Borisy GG. Cellular motility driven by assembly and disassembly of actin filaments. *Cell* 2003;**112**:453–65.

146. Levayer R, Lecuit T. Biomechanical regulation of contractility: spatial control and dynamics. *Trends Cell Biol* 2012;**22**:61–81.

147. Salbreux G, Charras G, Paluch E. Actin cortex mechanics and cellular morphogenesis. *Trends Cell Biol* 2012;**22**:536–45.

148. Bray D, White J. Cortical flow in animal cells. *Science* 1988;**239**:883–9.

149. Stewart MP, Helenius J, Toyoda Y, Ramanathan SP, Muller DJ, Hyman AA. Hydrostatic pressure and the actomyosin cortex drive mitotic cell rounding. *Nature* 2011;**469**:226–30.

150. Kumari S, Curado S, Mayya V, Dustin ML. T cell antigen receptor activation and actin cytoskeleton remodeling. *Biochim Biophys Acta* 2014;**1838**:546–56.

151. Pelham RJ, Chang F. Actin dynamics in the contractile ring during cytokinesis in fission yeast. *Nature* 2002;**419**:82–6.

152. Theriot JA. The polymerization motor. *Traffic* 2000;**1**:19–28.

153. Bovellan M, Romeo Y, Biro M, Boden A, Chugh P, Yonis A, Vaghela M, Fritzsche M, Moulding D, Thorogate R, et al. Cellular control of cortical actin nucleation. *Curr Biol* 2014;**24**:1628–35.

154. Fritzsche M, Lewalle A, Duke T, Kruse K, Charras G. Analysis of turnover dynamics of the submembranous actin cortex. *Mol Biol Cell* 2013;**24**:757–67.

155. Fritzsche M, Erlenkamper C, Moeendarbary E, Charras G, Kruse K. Actin kinetics shapes cortical network structure and mechanics. *Sci Adv* 2016;**2**:e1501337.

156. Zumdieck A, Kruse K, Bringmann H, Hyman AA, Jülicher F. Stress generation and filament turnover during actin ring constriction. *PLoS One* 2007;**2**:e696.

157. Koestler SA, Steffen A, Nemethova M, Winterhoff M, Luo N, Holleboom JM, Krupp J, Jacob S, Vinzenz M, Schur F, et al. Arp2/3 complex is essential for actin network treadmilling as well as for targeting of capping protein and cofilin. *Mol Biol Cell* 2013;**24**:2861–75.

158. Ilani T, Vasiliver-Shamis G, Vardhana S, Bretscher A, Dustin ML. T cell antigen receptor signaling and immunological synapse stability require myosin IIA. *Nat Immunol* 2009;**10**:531–9.

159. Malinova D, Fritzsche M, Nowosad CR, Armer H, Munro PM, Blundell MP, Charras G, Tolar P, Bouma G, Thrasher AJ. WASp-dependent actin cytoskeleton stability at the dendritic cell immunological synapse is required for extensive, functional T cell contacts. *J Leukoc Biol* 2016;**99**:699–710.

160. Bai M, Missel AR, Levine AJ, Klug WS. On the role of the filament length distribution in the mechanics of semiflexible networks. *Acta Biomater* 2011;**7**:2109–18.

161. Judokusumo E, Tabdanov E, Kumari S, Dustin ML, Kam LC. Mechanosensing in T lymphocyte activation. *Biophys J* 2012;**102**:L5–7.

162. Basu R, Whitlock BM, Husson J, Le Floc'h A, Jin W, Oyler-Yaniv A, Dotiwala F, Giannone G, Hivroz C, Biais N, et al. Cytotoxic T cells use mechanical force to potentiate target cell killing. *Cell* 2016;**165**:100–10.

163. Burroughs NJ, Lazic Z, van der Merwe PA. Ligand detection and discrimination by spatial relocalization: a kinase-phosphatase segregation model of TCR activation. *Biophys J* 2006;**91**:1619–29.

164. Colin-York H, Shrestha D, Felce JH, Waithe D, Moeendarbary E, Davis SJ, Eggeling C, Fritzsche M. Super-resolved traction force microscopy (STFM). *Nano Lett* 2016;**16**:2633–8.

165. Majstoravich S, Zhang J, Nicholson-Dykstra S, Linder S, Friedrich W, Siminovitch KA, Higgs HN. Lymphocyte microvilli are dynamic, actin-dependent structures that do not require Wiskott-Aldrich syndrome protein (WASp) for their morphology. *Blood* 2004;**104**:1396–403.

166. Harris ES, Gauvin TJ, Heimsath EG, Higgs HN. Assembly of filopodia by the formin FRL2 (FMNL3). *Cytoskeleton (Hoboken)* 2010;**67**:755–72.

167. Jung Y, Riven I, Feigelson SW, Kartvelishvily E, Tohya K, Miyasaka M, Alon R, Haran G. Three-dimensional localization of T-cell receptors in relation to microvilli using a combination of superresolution microscopies. *Proc Natl Acad Sci U S A* 2016;**113**:E5916–24.

168. Negulescu PA, Krasieva TB, Khan A, Kerschbaum HH, Cahalan MD. Polarity of T cell shape, motility, and sensitivity to antigen. *Immunity* 1996;**4**:421–30.

169. Wei X, Tromberg BJ, Cahalan MD. Mapping the sensitivity of T cells with an optical trap: polarity and minimal number of receptors for Ca(2+) signaling. *Proc Natl Acad Sci U S A* 1999;**96**:8471–6.

170. von Andrian UH, Hasslen SR, Nelson RD, Erlandsen SL, Butcher EC. A central role for microvillous receptor presentation in leukocyte adhesion under flow. *Cell* 1995;**82**:989–99.

171. Ivetic A, Florey O, Deka J, Haskard DO, Ager A, Ridley AJ. Mutagenesis of the ezrin-radixin-moesin binding domain of L-selectin tail affects shedding, microvillar positioning, and leukocyte tethering. *J Biol Chem* 2004;**279**:33263–72.

172. Peterson EJ, Woods ML, Dmowski SA, Derimanov G, Jordan MS, Wu JN, Myung PS, Liu QH, Pribila JT, Freedman BD, et al. Coupling of the TCR to integrin activation by Slap-130/Fyb. *Science* 2001;**293**:2263–5.

173. Crites TJ, Padhan K, Muller J, Krogsgaard M, Gudla PR, Lockett SJ, Varma R. TCR microclusters pre-exist and contain molecules necessary for TCR signal transduction. *J Immunol* 2014;**193**:56–67.

174. Lillemeier BF, Mortelmaier MA, Forstner MB, Huppa JB, Groves JT, Davis MM. TCR and Lat are expressed on separate protein islands on T cell membranes and concatenate during activation. *Nat Immunol* 2010;**11**:90–6.

175. Brodovitch A, Limozin L, Bongrand P, Pierres A. Use of TIRF to monitor T-lymphocyte membrane dynamics with submicrometer and subsecond resolution. *Cell Mol Bioeng* 2015;**8**:178–86.

176. Hashimoto-Tane A, Sakuma M, Ike H, Yokosuka T, Kimura Y, Ohara O, Saito T. Micro-adhesion rings surrounding TCR microclusters are essential for T cell activation. *J Exp Med* 2016;**213**:1609–25.

177. Mossman KD, Campi G, Groves JT, Dustin ML. Altered TCR signaling from geometrically repatterned immunological synapses. *Science* 2005;**310**:1191–3.

178. Kumari S, Vardhana S, Cammer M, Curado S, Santos L, Sheetz MP, Dustin ML. T lymphocyte myosin IIA is required for maturation of the immunological synapse. *Front Immunol* 2012;**3**:230.

179. Murugesan S, Hong J, Yi J, Li D, Beach JR, Shao L, Meinhardt J, Madison G, Wu X, Betzig E, Hammer JA. Formin-generated actomyosin arcs propel T cell receptor microcluster movement at the immune synapse. *J Cell Biol* 2016;**215**:383–99.

180. Hu S, Planus E, Georgess D, Place C, Wang X, Albiges-Rizo C, Jurdic P, Geminard JC. Podosome rings generate forces that drive saltatory osteoclast migration. *Mol Biol Cell* 2011;**22**:3120–6.

181. Labernadie A, Thibault C, Vieu C, Maridonneau-Parini I, Charriere GM. Dynamics of podosome stiffness revealed by atomic force microscopy. *Proc Natl Acad Sci U S A* 2010;**107**:21016–21.

182. van den Dries K, Schwartz SL, Byars J, Meddens MB, Bolomini-Vittori M, Lidke DS, Figdor CG, Lidke KA, Cambi A. Dual-color superresolution microscopy reveals nanoscale organization of mechanosensory podosomes. *Mol Biol Cell* 2013;**24**:2112–23.

183. Luxenburg C, Geblinger D, Klein E, Anderson K, Hanein D, Geiger B, Addadi L. The architecture of the adhesive apparatus of cultured osteoclasts: from podosome formation to sealing zone assembly. *PLoS One* 2007;**2**:e179.

184. Tu C, Ortega-Cava CF, Chen G, Fernandes ND, Cavallo-Medved D, Sloane BF, Band V, Band H. Lysosomal cathepsin B participates in the podosome-mediated extracellular matrix degradation and invasion via secreted lysosomes in v-Src fibroblasts. *Cancer Res* 2008;**68**:9147–56.

185. Panzer L, Trube L, Klose M, Joosten B, Slotman J, Cambi A, Linder S. The formins FHOD1 and INF2 regulate inter- and intra-structural contractility of podosomes. *J Cell Sci* 2016;**129**:298–313.

186. Barda-Saad M, Braiman A, Titerence R, Bunnell SC, Barr VA, Samelson LE. Dynamic molecular interactions linking the T cell antigen receptor to the actin cytoskeleton. *Nat Immunol* 2005;**6**:80–9.

187. Beemiller P, Jacobelli J, Krummel MF. Integration of the movement of signaling microclusters with cellular motility in immunological synapses. *Nat Immunol* 2012;**13**:787–95.

188. Dobereiner HG, Dubin-Thaler BJ, Hofman JM, Xenias HS, Sims TN, Giannone G, Dustin ML, Wiggins CH, Sheetz MP. Lateral membrane waves constitute a universal dynamic pattern of motile cells. *Phys Rev Lett* 2006;**97**:038102.

189. Ashdown GW, Cope A, Wiseman PW, Owen DM. Molecular flow quantified beyond the diffraction limit by spatiotemporal image correlation of structured illumination microscopy data. *Biophys J* 2014;**107**:L21–3.

190. Dustin ML. The immunological synapse. *Cancer Immunol Res* 2014;**2**:1023–33.

191. Jun JK, Hubler AH. Formation and structure of ramified charge transportation networks in an electromechanical system. *Proc Natl Acad Sci U S A* 2005;**102**:536–40.

192. Wulfing C, Sjaastad MD, Davis MM. Visualizing the dynamics of T cell activation: intracellular adhesion molecule 1 migrates rapidly to the T cell/B cell interface and acts to sustain calcium levels. *Proc Natl Acad Sci U S A* 1998;**95**:6302–7.

193. Blanchoin L, Boujemaa-Paterski R, Sykes C, Plastino J. Actin dynamics, architecture, and mechanics in cell motility. *Physiol Rev* 2014;**94**:235–63.

194. Roybal KT, Sinai P, Verkade P, Murphy RF, Wulfing C. The actin-driven spatiotemporal organization of T-cell signaling at the system scale. *Immunol Rev* 2013;**256**:133–47.

195. Suzuki J, Yamasaki S, Wu J, Koretzky GA, Saito T. The actin cloud induced by LFA-1-mediated outside-in signals lowers the threshold for T-cell activation. *Blood* 2007;**109**: 168–75.

196. Liang Y, Cucchetti M, Roncagalli R, Yokosuka T, Malzac A, Bertosio E, Imbert J, Nijman IJ, Suchanek M, Saito T, et al. The lymphoid lineage-specific actin-uncapping protein Rltpr is essential for costimulation via CD28 and the development of regulatory T cells. *Nat Immunol* 2013;**14**:858–66.

197. Britton GJ, Ambler R, Clark DJ, Hill EV, Tunbridge HM, McNally KE, Burton BR, Butterweck P, Sabatos-Peyton C, Hampton-O'Neil LA, et al. PKCtheta links proximal T cell and Notch signaling through localized regulation of the actin cytoskeleton. *eLife* 2017;**6**: e20003.

198. Balagopalan L, Barr VA, Kortum RL, Park AK, Samelson LE. Cutting edge: cell surface linker for activation of T cells is recruited to microclusters and is active in signaling. *J Immunol* 2013;**190**:3849–53.

199. Liu H, Rhodes M, Wiest DL, Vignali DA. On the dynamics of TCR:CD3 complex cell surface expression and downmodulation. *Immunity* 2000;**13**:665–75.

200. Bonello G, Blanchard N, Montoya MC, Aguado E, Langlet C, He HT, Nunez-Cruz S, Malissen M, Sanchez-Madrid F, Olive D, et al. Dynamic recruitment of the adaptor protein LAT: LAT exists in two distinct intracellular pools and controls its own recruitment. *J Cell Sci* 2004;**117**:1009–16.

201. Ehrlich LI, Ebert PJ, Krummel MF, Weiss A, Davis MM. Dynamics of p56lck translocation to the T cell immunological synapse following agonist and antagonist stimulation. *Immunity* 2002;**17**:809–22.

202. Geiger B, Rosen D, Berke G. Spatial relationships of microtubule-organizing centers and the contact area of cytotoxic T lymphocytes and target cells. *J Cell Biol* 1982;**95**:137–43.

203. Kupfer A, Dennert G. Reorientation of the microtubule-organizing center and the Golgi apparatus in cloned cytotoxic lymphocytes triggered by binding to lysable target cells. *J Immunol* 1984;**133**:2762–6.

204. Stinchcombe JC, Majorovits E, Bossi G, Fuller S, Griffiths GM. Centrosome polarization delivers secretory granules to the immunological synapse. *Nature* 2006;**443**:462–5.

205. Soares H, Henriques R, Sachse M, Ventimiglia L, Alonso MA, Zimmer C, Thoulouze MI, Alcover A. Regulated vesicle fusion generates signaling nanoterritories that control T cell activation at the immunological synapse. *J Exp Med* 2013;**210**:2415–33.

206. Finetti F, Paccani SR, Riparbelli MG, Giacomello E, Perinetti G, Pazour GJ, Rosenbaum JL, Baldari CT. Intraflagellar transport is required for polarized recycling of the TCR/CD3 complex to the immune synapse. *Nat Cell Biol* 2009;**11**:1332–9.

207. Finetti F, Patrussi L, Galgano D, Cassioli C, Perinetti G, Pazour GJ, Baldari CT. The small GTPase Rab8 interacts with VAMP-3 to regulate the delivery of recycling T-cell receptors to the immune synapse. *J Cell Sci* 2015;**128**:2541–52.

208. Finetti F, Patrussi L, Masi G, Onnis A, Galgano D, Lucherini OM, Pazour GJ, Baldari CT. Specific recycling receptors are targeted to the immune synapse by the intraflagellar transport system. *J Cell Sci* 2014;**127**:1924–37.

209. Larghi P, Williamson DJ, Carpier JM, Dogniaux S, Chemin K, Bohineust A, Danglot L, Gaus K, Galli T, Hivroz C. VAMP7 controls T cell activation by regulating the recruitment and phosphorylation of vesicular Lat at TCR-activation sites. *Nat Immunol* 2013;**14**:723–31.

210. de la Roche M, Ritter AT, Angus KL, Dinsmore C, Earnshaw CH, Reiter JF, Griffiths GM. Hedgehog signaling controls T cell killing at the immunological synapse. *Science* 2013;**342**:1247–50.

211. Purbhoo MA, Liu H, Oddos S, Owen DM, Neil MA, Pageon SV, French PM, Rudd CE, Davis DM. Dynamics of subsynaptic vesicles and surface microclusters at the immunological synapse. *Sci Signal* 2010;**3**:ra36.

212. Williamson DJ, Owen DM, Rossy J, Magenau A, Wehrmann M, Gooding JJ, Gaus K. Pre-existing clusters of the adaptor Lat do not participate in early T cell signaling events. *Nat Immunol* 2011;**12**:655–62.

213. Naramura M, Jang IK, Kole H, Huang F, Haines D, Gu H. c-Cbl and Cbl-b regulate T cell responsiveness by promoting ligand-induced TCR down-modulation. *Nat Immunol* 2002;**3**:1192–9.

214. Valitutti S, Muller S, Salio M, Lanzavecchia A. Degradation of T cell receptor (TCR)-CD3-zeta complexes after antigenic stimulation. *J Exp Med* 1997;**185**:1859–64.

215. Choudhuri K, Llodra J, Roth EW, Tsai J, Gordo S, Wucherpfennig KW, Kam LC, Stokes DL, Dustin ML. Polarized release of T-cell-receptor-enriched microvesicles at the immunological synapse. *Nature* 2014;**507**:118–23.

216. Mittelbrunn M, Gutierrez-Vazquez C, Villarroya-Beltri C, Gonzalez S, Sanchez-Cabo F, Gonzalez MA, Bernad A, Sanchez-Madrid F. Unidirectional transfer of microRNA-loaded exosomes from T cells to antigen-presenting cells. *Nat Commun* 2011;**2**:282.

217. Bache KG, Brech A, Mehlum A, Stenmark H. Hrs regulates multivesicular body formation via ESCRT recruitment to endosomes. *J Cell Biol* 2003;**162**:435–42.

218. Vardhana S, Choudhuri K, Varma R, Dustin ML. Essential role of ubiquitin and TSG101 protein in formation and function of the central supramolecular activation cluster. *Immunity* 2010;**32**:531–40.

219. Okoye IS, Coomes SM, Pelly VS, Czieso S, Papayannopoulos V, Tolmachova T, Seabra MC, Wilson MS. MicroRNA-containing T-regulatory-cell-derived exosomes suppress pathogenic T helper 1 cells. *Immunity* 2014;**41**:89–103.

220. Dustin ML. What counts in the immunological synapse? *Mol Cell* 2014;**54**:255–62.

221. Dustin ML. Help to go: T cells transfer CD40L to antigen-presenting B cells. *Eur J Immunol* 2017;**47**:31–4.

222. Gardell JL, Parker DC. CD40L is transferred to antigen-presenting B cells during delivery of T-cell help. *Eur J Immunol* 2017;**47**:41–50.

223. Bridgeman A, Maelfait J, Davenne T, Partridge T, Peng Y, Mayer A, Dong T, Kaever V, Borrow P, Rehwinkel J. Viruses transfer the antiviral second messenger cGAMP between cells. *Science* 2015;**349**:1228–32.

224. Poo WJ, Conrad L, Janeway Jr. CA. Receptor-directed focusing of lymphokine release by helper T cells. *Nature* 1988;**332**:378–80.

225. Beal AM, Anikeeva N, Varma R, Cameron TO, Vasiliver-Shamis G, Norris PJ, Dustin ML, Sykulev Y. Kinetics of early T cell receptor signaling regulate the pathway of lytic granule delivery to the secretory domain. *Immunity* 2009;**31**:632–42.

226. Stinchcombe J, Bossi G, Griffiths GM. Linking albinism and immunity: the secrets of secretory lysosomes. *Science* 2004;**305**:55–9.

227. Menager MM, Menasche G, Romao M, Knapnougel P, Ho CH, Garfa M, Raposo G, Feldmann J, Fischer A, de Saint Basile G. Secretory cytotoxic granule maturation and exocytosis require the effector protein hMunc13-4. *Nat Immunol* 2007;**8**:257–67.

228. Qu B, Pattu V, Junker C, Schwarz EC, Bhat SS, Kummerow C, Marshall M, Matti U, Neumann F, Pfreundschuh M, et al. Docking of lytic granules at the immunological synapse in human CTL requires Vti1b-dependent pairing with CD3 endosomes. *J Immunol* 2011;**186**:6894–904.

229. Peters PJ, Geuze HJ, van der Donk HA, Borst J. A new model for lethal hit delivery by cytotoxic T lymphocytes. *Immunol Today* 1990;**11**:28–32.

230. Peters PJ, Geuze HJ, Van der Donk HA, Slot JW, Griffith JM, Stam NJ, Clevers HC, Borst J. Molecules relevant for T cell-target cell interaction are present in cytolytic granules of human T lymphocytes. *Eur J Immunol* 1989;**19**:1469–75.

231. Dudenhoffer-Pfeifer M, Schirra C, Pattu V, Halimani M, Maier-Peuschel M, Marshall MR, Matti U, Becherer U, Dirks J, Jung M, et al. Different Munc13 isoforms function as priming factors in lytic granule release from murine cytotoxic T lymphocytes. *Traffic* 2013;**14**:798–809.

232. Marshall MR, Pattu V, Halimani M, Maier-Peuschel M, Muller ML, Becherer U, Hong W, Hoth M, Tschernig T, Bryceson YT, Rettig J. VAMP8-dependent fusion of recycling endosomes with the plasma membrane facilitates T lymphocyte cytotoxicity. *J Cell Biol* 2015;**210**:135–51.

233. Colin-York H, Eggeling C, Fritzsche M. Dissection of mechanical force in living cells by super-resolved traction force microscopy. *Nat Protoc* 2017;**12**:783–96.

234. Norcross MA. A synaptic basis for T-lymphocyte activation. *Ann Immunol (Paris)* 1984;**135D**:113–34.

235. Li D, Shao L, Chen BC, Zhang X, Zhang M, Moses B, Milkie DE, Beach JR, Hammer 3rd JA, Pasham M, et al. Advanced imaging. Extended-resolution structured illumination imaging of endocytic and cytoskeletal dynamics. *Science* 2015;**349**:aab3500.

Chapter 2

Principles of Protein Recognition by Small T-Cell Adhesion Proteins and Costimulatory Receptors

Shinji Ikemizu*, Simon J. Davis†

*Kumamoto University, Kumamoto, Japan, †University of Oxford, Oxford, United Kingdom

2.1 INTRODUCTION

The analysis of leukocyte cell surface molecules has yielded fundamental insights into immune phenomena. After it was demonstrated that perturbing these molecules could profoundly alter leukocyte behavior,[1] it seemed likely that opportunities for therapeutic intervention would also follow from a detailed understanding of how they function. This promise is now being abundantly fulfilled, most dramatically in the case of "immune checkpoint" blockade, which is transforming cancer medicine.[2]

A full understanding of the functions of leukocyte cell surface molecules would require knowing (i) which molecules are expressed, (ii) the general features of the structures and interactions of these proteins and how binding initiates cell activation in the case of signaling receptors, and (iii) how the molecules are organized and how local or global changes in their organization affect, if at all, their functions. The advent of monoclonal antibodies in the mid-1970s[3,4] revolutionized the analysis of the leukocyte cell surface by allowing the identification and isolation of low abundance species in complex mixtures of proteins. A survey we undertook over a decade ago[5] suggested that, at least in terms of immune function-related proteins, the composition of the T-cell surface could even then be considered to be solved. Although the extent to which changes in their organization mediate the functions of cell surface proteins is contested, it is clear that such rearrangements do take place on a variety of length scales.[6–8]

In the early 1990s, the structural basis of protein recognition at the leukocyte, or indeed any other cell surface, was poorly understood. Soluble forms

Structural Biology in Immunology. https://doi.org/10.1016/B978-0-12-803369-2.00002-4

of B-cell antigen receptors (i.e., Bence-Jones proteins and antibody Fab fragments) were the first leukocyte recognition structures solved,[9,10] and complexes of Fab fragments with their protein antigens subsequently contributed important insights into the general features of protein-protein recognition.[11,12] However, it was the iconic structure of the human class I major histocompatibility antigen, HLA-A2 (Ref. 13), with electron density trapped between two long α helices at the "top" of the molecule that was unaccounted for but had to comprise peptide fragments analogous to antigens "presented" by A2 to T-cell receptors (TCRs), that transformed our field, convincing even hardened immunologists of the remarkable explanatory power of structural biology. This was followed by structures of peptide/MHC class II (pMHC II),[14] as well as CD4 (Refs. 15,16) and CD8 (Ref. 17) proteins. At about this time, measurements of the affinities of these interactions started to reveal that binding is extremely weak, consistent with the requirement that leukocyte interactions are easily reversed.[18] This prompted the question: how can protein recognition be both weak and specific?

Obtaining the structures of cell surface proteins needed to answer this question was not a trivial matter, however. One problem was their complexity, with some of the key proteins comprising complexes of more than four polypeptides, for example, TCR/pMHC complexes. However, it seemed likely that good progress in understanding the principles of protein binding at the leukocyte cell surface could be achieved by studying simpler interacting proteins, ideally monomeric receptors that bound their monomeric ligands monovalently. To be representative, such pairs of proteins needed ideally to come from the immunoglobulin superfamily (IgSF), since this group of molecules is the most highly represented of all protein superfamilies at the cell surface.[19]

A second obstacle was the "glycosylation problem." Only crystallography could yield atomic-scale structures the size of complexed cell surface proteins and heterologous expression was required to produce the large amounts of protein needed for growing crystals. Since they were almost invariably glycoproteins, methods for deglycosylating the proteins were needed since N-glycosylation generally prevents the formation of reproducible lattice contacts in crystals, owing to its size, flexibility, and diversity. The most promising approach, it seemed to us, would involve deglycosylating the purified proteins rather than preventing sugar addition because cotranslational glycosylation is often required for correct protein folding. Our solution[20] involved arresting N-glycan processing at a postfolding, endoglycosidase (endo) H- or endo F1-sensitive, largely oligomannose stage using lectin-resistant Chinese hamster ovary (CHO)-derived cell lines (e.g., Lec3.2.8.1 cells[21]). These cells were deficient, most importantly, in glucose N-acetyltransferase 1, the enzyme that catalyzes the first essential step in building complex N-glycans from a seven-sugar endo H-sensitive oligomannose precursor. We complemented this approach first by adding the α-glucosidase I inhibitor N-butyldeoxynojirimycin (NB-DNJ) to Lec3.2.8.1 cell cultures,[22] and later by using the α-mannosidase I and II inhibitors kifunensine and swainsonine to block oligosaccharide processing in high-throughput mammalian expression systems utilizing human embryonic kidney 293T cells.[23] With relatively few exceptions, in our experience the poly-dispersity in solution of endo H/F1-treated proteins was indistinguishable from that of wild-type proteins, whereas glycoproteins completely deglycosylated with peptide:N-glycanase F, for example, tended to aggregate.[24]

Using these approaches, we set out to understand the principles of protein interactions at leukocyte surfaces. We focused first on interactions of CD2 with its ligands, which are small IgSF adhesion proteins comprising single poly-peptide chains producible in large quantities, and then on similar small "co-stimulatory" signaling proteins including CD28, CTLA-4, and PD-1. Here we summarize what we learnt from the structural analysis of these proteins.

2.2   CELL-CELL RECOGNITION AND ADHESION: CD2 FAMILY PROTEINS

The CD2 family of proteins comprises a subset of the IgSF, made up of mainly small hematopoietic cell-cell recognition proteins. The proteins are encoded in two clusters of genes that are located on human chromosome 1, on each side of the centromere. The archetypal proteins, CD2 and CD58 (also known as LFA-3), are encoded on the p arm, and the q arm encodes nine more proteins, that is, BLAME, SF2001 (CD2F10), NTB-A (SF2000), CD84, CD150 (SLAM), CD48, CS1 (19A, CRACC), CD229 (Ly9), and CD244 (2B4; reviewed in Ref. 25). CD2 and CD58 were the first two proteins shown to mediate heterophilic adhesion,[26,27] serving as a paradigm for adhesive interactions within the IgSF. Attempts to identify a murine homologue of CD58 eventually led instead to the finding that mouse and rat CD2 bind a different molecule, CD48 (Ref. 28).

CD2 delivers mitogenic signals to T cells, especially in the presence of cer-tain combinations of anti-CD2 antibodies,[29] albeit in a strictly TCR-dependent manner.[30] The phenotypes of CD2-deficient mice revealed that the CD2/CD48 interaction is not essential for apparently normal immunity.[31] Instead, CD2 has the subtler role of "fine tuning" the T-cell repertoire by setting thresholds for T-cell activation.[32] In contrast, T-cell activation in mice deficient in CD48 ex-pressed on hematopoietic cells was severely impaired,[33] suggesting that CD48 does not only bind CD2. This is now explained by the finding that CD48 also binds CD244 (Ref. 34). CD244 is expressed on NK cells and a subset of T cells, where it triggers the nonmajor histocompatibility complex (MHC)-restricted killing of CD48-expressing target cells.[35] The structure of the mouse homo-logue of CD244 has now been determined using NMR methods.[36] Six of the q-arm encoded proteins carry the tyrosine phosphorylation motif, Thr-Ile/Val-Tyr-Xaa-Xaa-Val/Ile, that binds the SLAM-associated protein, SAP, implicated in X-linked lymphoproliferative disease.[37] The CD2 subset of the IgSF likely comprises a network of interactions that is mostly uncharacterized beyond those involving CD2 and CD48. It has been proposed that several of the q-arm en-coded proteins are homophilic (Ref. 25), like SLAM.[38]

Sequence analysis predicted that the extracellular regions of CD2, CD58, and CD48 consist of two IgSF domains, with the first lacking a canonical disulfide bond, as confirmed by NMR analysis of rat CD2 domain 1 (d1).[39] Ligand binding activity was known to reside in d1 of CD2 (Ref. 40), with mutational data[41] reinterpreted in light of the structure directly implicating the GFCC′C″ β-sheet. Even before the advent of Biacore™ technology, the affinity of the CD2/CD58 interaction seemed to be low ($2 \times 10^6 M^{-1}$; Ref. 42). The chromosomal organization of their genes pointed to CD2 family proteins having evolved from a common precursor[43,44] proposed to have been homophilic.[45] It was even predicted[46] that the twofold rotational symmetry of a primordial homophilic interaction would be preserved in evolution for the heterotypic binding of CD2 to CD58. It was suggested that, analogous to the dimerization of antibody variable domains, the CD2/CD58 interaction would involve equivalent β-sheets.[46]

2.2.1 Rat sCD2 (1992)

Rat (r) soluble (s) CD2 was the first test of the approach of expressing glycoproteins for crystallization under conditions in which N-glycan processing was manipulated in order to mitigate the detrimental effects of glycosylation on crystallization.[20] Work on rsCD2 produced the first complete structure of the extracellular region of a cell adhesion molecule.[47] A large lattice contact observed in the crystals offered a first glimpse of the types of complexes these proteins would form and a putative model for the primordial homophilic interaction.

2.2.1.1 The Structure

rsCD2 was expressed in CHO-derived Lec3.2.8.1 cells,[21] resulting in a secreted glycoprotein with oligosaccharides (predominantly $Man_5GlcNAc_2$) amenable to deglycosylation with endo H.[20] Endo H-deglycosylated rsCD2 readily formed crystals belonging to space group $P4_12_12$ with unit cell dimensions $a = b = 111.4 Å$, $c = 86.9 Å$, which diffracted to Bragg spacings of 2.5 Å.[47] Multiple isomorphous replacement, phase improvement and extension by solvent-flattening, and a single round of twofold density averaging yielded unambiguous electron density. The crystals contained two rsCD2 molecules per asymmetric unit. Owing to differences in what turned out to be hinge bending, the domains of each molecule were separately restrained to obey noncrystallographic symmetry during refinement.

The extracellular domain (ECD) of rat CD2, as anticipated,[48] consisted of two domains with antiparallel β-sheets comprising an IgSF fold.[47] At the time, the most similar structure was the NH_2-terminal two-domain fragment of CD4 (CD4d1d2; Refs. 15,16). In rat CD2, as in CD4d1d2, the domains abutted, producing a rod-like molecule with dimensions of $\sim 20 \times \sim 25 \times \sim 75 Å^3$. In contrast to CD4d1d2, d1 and d2 of rat CD2 were joined by a four-residue linker. The overall structural arrangement resulted in the d1 GFCC′C″ β-sheet comprising a highly accessible platform $\sim 75 Å$ above the cell surface (Fig. 2.1A).

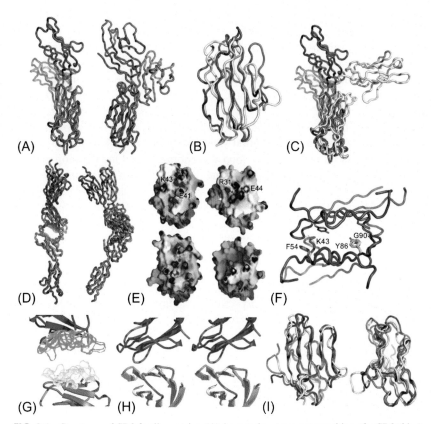

FIG. 2.1 Structures of CD2 family proteins. (A) An α-carbon trace superposition of rsCD2 (*blue*) and human CD4d1d2 (*red*), in two orthogonal views. The molecules are superimposed on CD2 d2 using SHP.[49] (B) An α-carbon backbone superposition of rat CD2 d1 (residues 2-99; *blue*) and the VH domain of antibody REI (residues 1-114; *white*). (C) An α-carbon trace superposition of rsCD2 (*blue*), human CD4d1d2 (*red*), and Fab NEW light chain (*white*). The molecules are matched on CD2 d2. (D) Two orthogonal views of α-carbon trace superpositions of the two versions of the homophilic interaction observed in crystals of rsCD2. Copy 1 molecules are colored *blue*; copy 2 molecules are colored *red*. Superposition is on domain 1 of the *blue* molecule. (E) The ligand binding surfaces of domain 1 of rat CD2 (*top left*), rat CD48 (*top right*), human CD2 (*bottom left*), and CD58 (*bottom right*), colored according to the native electrostatic potential of the surfaces calculated at neutral pH. Contours are at ±8.5 kT (*blue* positive, *red* negative). Residues mutated when analyzing the electrostatic basis of binding specificity[50] are labeled. (F) A close-up of the interacting GFCC'C" faces of the homophilic contact observed in the hsCD2 crystals. Main chain hydrogen (H)-bonds between Gly90 and Lys43 observed at the homophilic contact in the crystals of hsCD2 (*red dashed lines*) are superimposed on the Cα backbone of human CD2 d1 (*blue*). Side chains of Phe54 and Tyr86 (*red*) of human CD2 d1 and its symmetry-related partner are displayed in stick format. The equivalent residues and H-bonds for copies 1 and 2 of the homophilic contact observed in the rsCD2 crystals are superimposed (colored *green* and *yellow*, respectively). (G) Structures of the interacting surfaces of human CD2 (*blue*) and CD58 (*red*) following "undocking" of the proteins by 5–10Å, revealing the very poor shape complementarity at the binding sites (shown semitransparently). (H) Comparison of the complex of human CD2 (*blue*) and CD58 (*red*) that was predicted to form by maximizing electrostatic potential at the interface (*left*), with the actual, native complex subsequently determined by Wang et al.[51] (I) An α-carbon backbone superposition of rat CD2 d1 (residues 2-99; *blue*), rat CD48 d1 (residues 1-98; *red*), and mouse CD244 d1 (residues 1-114; *white*).

The topology of d1 was that of an IgSF V-set domain, that is, two sheets of β-strands conventionally labeled DEB and AGFCC'C". Despite lacking the usual disulfide, the positions of all the β-strands in the V-set domain framework were conserved. However, of the loops, only the AB and EF loops had similar conformations in d1 of rat CD2 and CD4, and the Vκ variable (V) domain of the Bence-Jones protein REI (Fig. 2.1B). As in CD4, the C'C" loop was longer than in antibody V domains, but unlike CD4, the orientation maintained the flat surface of the β-sheet. In addition, whereas the CC' and FG loops mediating antibody V-domain dimerization were shortened in CD4 relative to those in antibodies, in rat CD2 the CC' loop was shortened and the FG loop greatly lengthened. Although conserved β-bulges in the C' and G β-strands thought to be important for V-domain homodimerization[52] were absent, β-bulges were positioned in rat CD2 d1 immediately after the CC' and FG β-turns, limiting the characteristic twist to the tips of these loops.

At the end of d1 β-strand G in rat CD2, the main chain continued in an extended conformation for four residues held at the edge of the d2 β-sandwich by H-bonds to both β-sheets, before forming a standard β-strand A in d2. This "loosened" the tightly abutting domain junction seen in CD4d1d2 by sliding d2 down by four residues with respect to d1, adding ~15Å to the length of the protein (Fig. 2.1A). The d1/d2 interface, ~400Å^2 in total buried surface area, was much smaller than that buried in CD4d1d2 (880Å^2). As in CD4d1d2, rat CD2 d1 and d2 were related by a rotation of ~160 degrees about the long axis of the molecule, but a tilt of some 45 degrees from this axis was required for d1 superposition. The domain orientations of rat CD2 and CD4d1d2 were both very different from those in immunoglobulins (Fig. 2.1C). Slight changes in main-chain torsion angles in the linker generated substantial (7 degrees) hinge-bending shifts in domain orientation for the two copies of rsCD2, and more flexibility was expected in vivo.

As predicted by Williams and Barclay on the basis of sequence comparisons alone,[45] d2 of rat CD2 had both antibody V- and constant (C)-domain like character, justifying its inclusion in the C2-set of the IgSF. Superpositioning gave good matches to d2 of CD4 and to an antibody C domain, and also produced a very striking fit in the region of the G, F, C, and C' β-strands to d1 of rat CD2, emphasizing the evolutionary relatedness of all these domains. Two disulfide bonds in rat CD2 were also as predicted, with Cys117 and Cys157 forming the "canonical" IgSF disulfide, and Cys110 and Cys174 linking the ends of the A and G β-strands and tethering the protein to a short C-terminal stalk leading to the membrane. The base of d2 was neutrally charged, suggesting that it might not directly contact the cell surface. The only conserved glycosylation site in human and rat CD2 (Asn112) placed glycosylation at the bottom of d2, where it could have influenced the "posture" of the molecule.

Of the contacts in the crystal, one that packed rsCD2 molecules related by twofold rotational symmetry (Fig. 2.1D) was notable for its large area (650–690Å^2 buried/molecule) and intimacy. It was especially striking that both copies of rsCD2 formed this association. Given that it was mediated by the d1 GFCC′C″ β-sheet, specifically the CC′ and FG loops, the association had some similarity to antibody V-domain dimerization, although there were also important differences. Antibody V-domains dimerize via a specialized "three-layer" interaction[52] dependent on the extensive twist induced by the C′ and G strand β-bulges. Positioning the equivalent β-bulges at the ends of the CC′ and FG loops in rat CD2 limited the extent of the twist, and because the loops also had different lengths, the rsCD2 association depended on main-chain H-bonding at the tips of the CC′ and FG loops and direct interactions between the residues on the GFCC′C″ β-sheets. The angle between the respective β-sheets therefore differed radically (by ~60 degrees) from the characteristic angle observed for V domains (50 degrees). As such, the rsCD2 interaction most closely resembled the standard orthogonal class of β-sheet packing. Mutational analyses of human CD2 (Ref. 41) implied that the CD58 binding site spanned the diagonally opposed CC′ and FG loops of the GFCC′C″ β-sheet. The equivalent surface in rat CD2, walled in on either side by the CC′ and FG loops, was carpeted with assorted charged side chains, giving an electrostatically variegated but rather flat surface (Fig. 2.1E, top left).

2.2.1.2 What We Learnt

a. Comparisons with CD4d1d2 highlighted several important structure-function relationships for CD2 as a small adhesion protein. First, a degree of orientational flexibility provided by the interdomain linker and the C-terminal stalk in CD2 likely facilitates docking with molecules on opposing cell surfaces. Second, despite having slightly fewer residues, CD2 was markedly longer than CD4d1d2, increasing exposure of the putative ligand-binding d1 GFCC′C″ β-sheet. This effect was magnified by a third difference between CD2 and CD4d1d2, that is, the tilt of d1 that positioned this β-sheet roughly parallel with the cell surface. Flexibility and the location of ligand-binding sites close to the top of adhesion molecules were predicted to feature generally in their organization.

b. It had been proposed that the adhesion function of IgSF proteins predated their involvement in antigen recognition.[45] The presence of a homophilic interaction as the dominant contact in the rsCD2 crystals lent support to the notion[46] that the interaction of antibody V-domains (through their GFCC′C″ β-sheets) originated as a homophilic association having twofold rotational symmetry. However, the rsCD2 association exhibited several differences from standard V-domain dimerization, offering a new paradigm for adhesive interactions. We proposed that, in particular, the position of β-bulge conformations in the C′ and G β-strands and the lengths of the CC′ and FG loops, combined with the effects of the linker on the geometry of dimerization, allowed a switch from a dimerization mode suitable for intermolecular adhesion to the intramolecular version observed in the Fabs of antibodies.

c. The epitopes of several monoclonal antibodies raised against human CD2 had been mapped to three discrete regions.[41] Region 1 and 2 antibodies bound opposite corners of the GFCC'C" β-sheet of d1 and blocked ligand interactions, whereas region 1 or 2 antibodies paired with region 3 antibodies, which bind to the CC' loop in d2, were known to activate T cells. It had been proposed[29] that enhanced region 3 antibody binding following T-cell activation or in the presence of d1 antibodies relied on a conformational rearrangement in d1, but the new structural data argued strongly against this.

2.2.2 Human sCD2 (1994)

Comparison of the sequences of human, rat, mouse, and equine CD2 had implied that several previously unique features of CD2 were conserved and functionally important.[53] To confirm these predictions, the crystal structure of human (h) sCD2 was determined.[54] This proved worthwhile as many of the important structural features notable in rat CD2 were reprised or exaggerated in the human structure.

2.2.2.1 The Structure

The ECD of human CD2 was expressed in CHO cells in the presence of the glucosidase I inhibitor, NB-DNJ. NB-DNJ use broadened the approach of altering oligosaccharide processing and was effective because these cells lack a salvage pathway that would have restored full processing.[22] Deglycosylated hsCD2 readily formed crystals diffracting to 2.5 Å that belonged to space group $P3_121$ with unit cell dimensions of $a = b = 88.3$ Å, $c = 51.3$ Å, $\alpha = \beta = 90$ degrees, $\gamma = 120$ degrees. The structure was determined using single isomorphous replacement including anomalous scattering data after attempts at molecular replacement proved fruitless and it had been noticed that sites binding mercury in rsCD2 were probably conserved in human CD2. Human sCD2 was comprised of two antiparallel β-sandwich IgSF domains connected by a linker, with dimensions of $25 \times 30 \times 90$ Å^3 (Ref. 54). The overall structure of hsCD2 was very similar to that of rsCD2. The largest differences in secondary structure occurred in domain 2, for which H-bonding between β-strands F and G was extended for four pairs of residues in human CD2. The structural cores of d1 and d2 were well conserved and also structurally similar to domains of the same subset present in other IgSF proteins. The residues with the largest structural deviations in d1 were located in the BC and C'C" loops. A change in conformation in the BC loop was probably the result of a crystal contact causing a rigid-body shift over the whole loop. It had been proposed that this loop required intact glycosylation for structural stability,[55,56] but as also observed for deglycosylated rsCD2, the electron density for the BC loop in hsCD2 was relatively well defined. Human CD2 lacked the classic V-domain β-bulge sequence motif and instead contained the modified version immediately after the CC' and FG β-turns first observed for rat CD2. NMR structures of rat[39] and human[55] CD2 d1 confirmed that the β-bulges also formed in solution.

The human CD2 interdomain orientation angle differed by 13 degrees vs one copy of the rsCD2 crystal structure and by 20 degrees vs the other despite the sequence of these regions being highly conserved,[53] confirming that the linker of CD2 is inherently flexible. The linker of human CD2 was stabilized by hydrophobic contacts and a H-bond network in d2 involving residues whose ϕ,ψ angles differed for the most part by 7 degrees or less from the rat structure. These relatively subtle conformational differences appeared to be amplified by the rod-like nature of the molecule, giving the large shifts in orientations of d1 and d2. For both structures, the extended linker was considered to prevent the intimate association of the two IgSF domains, allowing flexibility in the orientation of the ligand-binding face with respect to the cell surface, an apparently unique feature of CD2.

Mutational analysis of human CD2 had identified the d1 GFCC'C" face as the ligand-binding site.[41,57,58] This surface was unusual as a site of protein-protein recognition for several reasons. First, it was relatively flat: the average distance of surface atoms from the least-squares plane defining it was ~1.8 Å. For rat CD2, this distance was ~1.6 Å, for CD4 d1 ~2.2 Å, for CD8 ~2.7 Å, and for the VL domain of Fab NEW ~4.5 Å.[54] Second, the surface was unusually highly charged (Fig. 2.1E, bottom left). Whereas most protein-protein recognition sites are compositionally similar to that of the average protein surface, that is, ~20% charged, ~25% polar, and ~55% nonpolar,[59] the solvent accessible area of the GFCC'C" face of human CD2 was 70% charged, 20% polar, and 10% nonpolar (35% charged, 35% polar, and 30% nonpolar for rat CD2). Since only 2 of 14 charged residues on this face of human CD2 were identical and 3 conservatively substituted vs rat CD2, and both these surfaces were relatively flat, we predicted that the distribution of charges would underpin the distinct ligand-binding specificities of the two proteins.

Unexpectedly, the head-to-head interaction involving the GFCC'C" faces of two pairs of symmetry-related molecules in the asymmetric unit of rsCD2 crystals[47] was reprised in the hsCD2 crystal lattice, despite the significant differences in the composition of the interacting surfaces and distinct space groups. The relative orientation of the interacting domains differed only 3 degrees from one of the two associations observed in the rsCD2 crystals (which had differed by 18 degrees). There was also considerable overlap between the residues buried in the lattice interaction and those implicated in ligand binding by CD2. The interface was large (~800 Å²/molecule) and also sufficiently well packed to completely exclude water. Gly90, Tyr86, and Phe54 in d1 seemed likely to have important roles in ligand-binding by CD2 since (i) each residue was involved in similar interactions in all three sets of head-to-head associations (Fig. 2.1F), and (ii) for highly exposed residues, they were unusually well conserved (identical in the four homologues sequenced at the time[53]). Moreover, because (i) main-chain H-bonding had a significant role in the interaction observed in the rsCD2 crystals, which was made possible by the β-bulges at the ends of the CC' and FG loops, (ii) the apolar nature of the residues forming the β-bulges was highly conserved (i.e., residues 39, 40, and 88, 89, rat CD2 numbering[53]), and (iii) H-bonds in the region of the β-bulges also formed in the hsCD2 lattice contact, it was predicted that main-chain H-bonding would contribute to the physiological interaction of CD2 with its ligands.

2.2.2.2 What We Learnt

a. Comparison of the structures of human and rat sCD2 suggested that, in addition to flexibility in the short peptide connecting the extracellular and the transmembrane domains, the key region of CD2 circumventing the restrictions on ligand binding imposed by membrane attachment was the conserved, flexible linker joining d1 and d2.

b. Contacts involving the ligand-binding faces of crystallographically related hsCD2 molecules recapitulated those already seen in rsCD2 crystals. The conserved features of these contacts were expected to mimic those involving native ligands and perhaps the interactions of other CD2-family proteins in vivo. Accordingly, it was predicted that ligand binding would involve main-chain H-bonding of residues adjacent to diagonally opposed, conserved CC′ and FG loop β-bulges in the GFCC′C″ face, including a conserved glycine, and side-chain interactions of conserved Tyr and Phe residues.

c. Assuming the contact mimicked native interactions, the area of the interface was comparable to that of previously characterized protein-protein interactions.[59] However, the affinity of CD2 for its ligands was known to be 10^4- to 10^5-fold lower than that of these more typical interactions due mostly to differences in off-rates,[18,59] allowing T cells to disengage from highly multivalent contacts with target cells. We argued that the unique features of the ligand-binding site of CD2, that is, its relative flatness and the large fraction of charged residues located there (particularly in the case of human CD2), ensured that ligand binding would have a large electrostatic component, in marked contrast to typical protein-protein interactions, which were highly dependent on hydrophobic contacts.[59]

2.2.3 The Role of Charged Residues in Ligand Binding by CD2 (1998)

The most remarkable feature of CD2 interactions was their very low affinities.[60,61] Subsequent studies of the interactions of B7-1 (Ref. 62) and CD62L[63] with their respective ligands implied that low affinities and very fast binding kinetics were general features of the interactions of leukocyte cell surface proteins. We used mutagenesis experiments and an analysis of the effects of ionic strength on CD2/CD48 binding to explore the link between the unusual structural properties of the ligand-binding face of CD2, that is, its flatness and high density of charged residues, and its ability to mediate weak specific protein recognition.[50]

2.2.3.1 Mutational Analysis of Rat CD2

In the absence of a structure of the rat CD2/CD48 complex, the ligand-binding GFCC'C" β-sheet of rat CD2 d1 was first mutated exhaustively to determine the extent of the CD48-binding site. The effects of 23 substitutions "drastically" altering the chemical properties of solvent-exposed residues were tested using surface plasmon resonance (SPR) as implemented in the Biacore™. Mutations of eight charged or polar residues (D28, E29, R31, E33, E41, K43, T86, and R87), two aromatic residues (Y81 and F49), and a single aliphatic residue (L38) disrupted ligand binding, suggesting that these residues, which comprised a contiguous surface extending diagonally from the FG loop to the CC' loop and included F, C, C', and C" β-strand residues, formed the ligand-binding site of rat CD2. The surface corresponded to the conserved contacts seen in rat and human sCD2 crystals[47,54] and with line-width perturbations and chemical shifts observed in two-dimensional NMR spectra of CD2 d1 recorded in the presence of sCD48 (Ref. 64).

The energetic contribution of each of the 11 residues was measured by substituting each residue with alanine. Substitutions of five of the eight charged or polar residues forming the binding site lead only to modest increases (<fourfold) or slight decreases (<twofold) in binding affinity. Twenty-fold or greater decreases in affinity were observed at only six positions: D28, E29, R31, L38, F49, and Y81, suggesting that, of all the charged residues, only D28, E29, and R31 participated in electrostatically favorable interactions. However, if these residues had contributed significantly to binding energy, the interaction ought to have been sensitive to electrostatic screening at high salt concentrations (0.05M to 2M NaCl), but it was instead observed to be completely unaffected.[50] Unless there were balancing favorable and unfavorable interactions involving D28, E29, and R31, we concluded that only 3 of 11 residues forming the ligand-binding site of CD2, that is, L38, F49, and Y81, provide most of the energy for ligand binding.

The possibility that charged residues in the ligand-binding site of CD2 might confer ligand-binding specificity was tested by examining the effects on specificity of mutating E41 and K43 to alanine. Complementary mutagenesis had shown that E41 and K43 of CD2 interact with the oppositely charged residues R31 and E44 of CD48, respectively[65] (see Fig. 2.1E). Whereas wild-type CD2 only bound strongly to wild-type CD48 and one mutant of CD48, the E41A and K43A mutants of CD2 tolerated both wild-type CD48 and a series of nine nonconservative substitutions at R31 or E44 of CD48, indicating that E41 and K43 of CD2 contribute to the specificity of recognition but not to the ligand-binding energy.[50]

2.2.3.2 What We Learnt

a. This first energetic analysis of low-affinity recognition at the cell surface suggested that interactions involving two aromatics and one aliphatic residue generated enough energy for weak ligand binding by CD2, and that eight charged or polar residues completing the flat ligand-binding site conferred a high degree of specificity without further increasing the binding affinity.

b. As this study was being completed, others[66] proposed that electrostatic interactions (including salt bridges) may generally confer specificity to protein-protein interactions and protein folding without necessarily being energetically favorable. This was because charged residues interact favorably with polar solvents such as water and the burial of these residues upon ligand binding requires disruption of these favorable interactions (desolvation). This unfavorable effect would be offset if these residues participated in electrostatically favorable interactions in the complex, but the net result would often be energetically neutral. We suggested that electrostatic complementarity could have special utility in low-affinity interactions because, unlike surface-shape complementarity, it allowed specificity and affinity to be uncoupled. This contrasted with the paradigm that emerged from the analysis of high-affinity interactions in which specificity and affinity were each dependent on the surface-shape complementarity of relatively hydrophobic surfaces.[59]

2.2.4   CD58 d1 (1999)

Antibodies reactive with CD2 and CD58 were among the first found to block human T-cell functions in vitro.[27] The cognate relationship of CD2 and CD58, the first heterophilic protein interaction identified at the cell surface, was established when Hünig showed that purified CD2 bound directly to cellular CD58 (Ref. 26). The mutational analysis of rat CD2 suggested an explanation for the unusual structural properties of the ligand-binding face of CD2 insofar as energetically neutral interactions involving charged residues in the ligand-binding region seemed to ensure that ligand recognition by CD2 was both weak and specific.[50] Analysis of the crystal structure of the CD2-binding domain of CD58 (Ref. 67) offered another test of this idea.

2.2.4.1   The Structure

In contrast to CD2, attempts to crystallize the deglycosylated ECD of CD58 expressed in the presence of NB-DNJ alone or in complex with hsCD2 were unsuccessful. Sequence alignment suggested that extended AB loops in d2 of each of the non-CD2 members of the CD2 subset of the IgSF might interfere with crystallization. The alignments also revealed a high degree of "linker" conservation among CD2-related proteins, implying that the ligand-binding domains of CD2 subset proteins might be interchangeable. A crystallizable, chimeric form of CD58 (cCD58), consisting of d1 of CD58 and d2 of rat CD2, readily formed crystals yielding diffraction data to Bragg spacings of 1.8 Å.[22] The crystals belonged to space group $P3_221$, with unit cell dimensions of $a = b = 118.1$ Å, $c = 52.1$ Å, $\alpha = \beta = 90$ degrees, $\gamma = 120$ degrees. The structure was solved by molecular replacement using rsCD2 as a search model.[67]

cCD58 resembled rat and human sCD2, while also diverging significantly. The conformation of the interdomain linker was completely conserved, with the principal contacts formed with residues in β-strand A and the AB loop of rat CD2 d1 W7GAL being duplicated in the chimera for CD58 d1 residues Y6GVV. The distinctive head-to-head lattice contacts formed by rat and human sCD2 (Refs. 47,54) were absent from the crystals of cCD58, likely owing to the large net negative charge of this face in CD58. Like CD2 d1, CD58 d1 had standard IgSF V-set AGFCC′C″/DEB domain topology. Consistent with having arisen by gene duplication, the structures of the cores of CD58 and CD2 d1 were very similar and, like CD2, CD58 d1 lacked the canonical β-strand B and E disulfide bond. Other similarities were the distinctive orientation of the C″ β-strand, the general lack of twist of the AGFCC′C″ β-sheet, and the shortened DE loop. Differences included truncation of the FG loop in CD58 and the absence of the characteristic β-bulge at the "top" of β-strand G.

Mutation of the d1 C, C′, and G β-strands, and the CC′ and FG loops identified the AGFCC′C″ β-sheet as the ligand-binding site of CD58 (Refs. 68,69). As such, the d1 AGFCC′C″ β-sheet of CD58 had two important features. First, and unexpectedly, whereas the surfaces of the equivalent β-sheets of rat and human CD2 were both flat, CD58 d1 had depressions between the F and G, and the C and C′ β-strands. The average distance of surface atoms from the least-squares plane defining the AGFCC′C″ β-sheet was ~3 Å for cCD58 vs 1.6–1.8 Å for rat and human CD2. There was therefore little or no shape complementarity in the ligand-binding sites of CD2 and CD58 (Fig. 2.1G). Second, and as anticipated,[68] charged residues were concentrated in the AGFCC′C″ β-sheet of CD58: 16 of 22 such residues in d1 were surface-exposed on this β-sheet, and, of these, 10 were acidic giving the ligand-binding site of CD58 a high degree of electrostatic complementarity to the more basic CD58-binding site of human CD2 (Fig. 2.1E, bottom right). The likely dependence of binding on electrostatic complementarity afforded an opportunity to predict the topology of binding (Fig. 2.1H). Without altering their unliganded side-chain conformations, using the human sCD2 crystal lattice contact as a template for "docking" human CD2 and CD58 generated five contacts between oppositely charged residues ($K34_{CD58}$-$D31_{CD2}$, $E37_{CD58}$-$R48_{CD2}$, $E39_{CD58}$-$R48_{CD2}$, $E42_{CD58}$-$K51_{CD2}$, and $E78_{CD58}$-$K34_{CD2}$) and one unfavorable interaction of residues with the same charge ($R44_{CD58}$-$R48_{CD2}$). In contrast, docking human CD2 and CD58 using homodimeric interactions of CD8α V-set domains[17] or the antiparallel homodimeric lattice contacts of P0 crystals[70] generated only one complementary interaction or a single, unfavorable contact, respectively. In addition, the total areas buried in CD8α- and P0-based complexes were only 68 and 49% of the areas buried in the complex modeled on sCD2 lattice contacts ($1638 Å^2$). Overall, these considerations suggested that native human CD2/CD58 complexes would be very similar to the homophilic interaction observed in sCD2 crystals.[67]

2.2.4.2 What We Learnt

a. The clustering of charged residues at their ligand-binding d1 AGFCC′C″ β-sheets implied that electrostatic contacts have a major role in CD2 binding to CD58. The topology of binding therefore was predicted to be the arrangement that generated the highest degree of electrostatic complementarity, buried the largest number of residues implicated by mutagenesis in binding, and occluded the largest overall surface area (as was confirmed when the actual structure of the native complex was published shortly after our structure of cCD58 (Ref. 51)).

b. The uncomplexed ligand-binding surfaces of human CD2 and CD58 exhibited little shape complementarity. Irrespective of the topology of binding, without major structural rearrangements, it was difficult to envisage how the depressions in the surface of the AGFCC'C" β-sheet of CD58 would be filled by CD2. Although the fit could have been somewhat better in vivo, it was expected that poor complementarity would in part be responsible for the low affinity of human CD2 for CD58. Poor shape complementarity was also a feature of the first structures of low affinity human and mouse TCR/peptide-MHC class I complexes.[71,72] We predicted that shape mismatches would frequently contribute to weak protein interactions at cell-cell contacts and that for these interactions, electrostatic complementarity would be the major or only source of binding specificity.

2.2.5 CD48 d1 (2006)

The binding of rat CD48 with CD2 differs from the interaction of human CD2 with CD58 insofar as it is weaker (four- to fivefold), and part of a broader network of interactions exhibiting cross-reactivity, that is, involving CD244 (2B4) and 2B4R. An NMR-based structural analysis of mouse CD244 had been published by others.[36] The structure of d1 of rat CD48 (Ref. 73) therefore completed the initial characterization of the murine CD2/CD244/CD48 receptor-ligand system and allowed structural comparisons with human CD2 and CD58. A complementary thermodynamic analysis went on to reveal unexpected differences in the mechanism of ligand binding by rat vs human CD2 (Refs. 73,74).

2.2.5.1 The Structure

Deglycosylated rat sCD48 did not crystallize alone, and although it crystallized very readily as a complex with rsCD2, the crystals did not diffract (SJD, unpublished data). Following the success of cCD58, CD48 d1 was expressed as a chimeric protein with rat CD2 d2 (cCD48) in Lec3.2.8.1 cells in the presence of NB-DNJ.[22] Over a period of 12 months, deglycosylated cCD48 formed crystals of sufficient size to produce X-ray diffraction data to Bragg spacings of 2.6 Å at a microfocus beamline. The crystals belonged to space group $I4_122$, with unit cell dimensions $a=b=96.78$ Å, $c=126.62$ Å. The structure was solved by molecular replacement using the coordinates of rat CD2 d2.

Structurally, cCD48 was, as expected, very similar to rsCD2 (Ref. 47) and cCD58 (Ref. 67). Modest differences included a slight increase in the "uprightness" of d1 of cCD48: by ~3 degrees vs cCD58, and ~5 degrees compared to

CD2. Otherwise, conservation of the residues interacting in the linker suggested that the ECD of CD48 would have the same topology as that of rat CD2, with the ligand-binding surface positioned close to the "top" of the molecule. cCD48, like cCD58, did not form the distinctive lattice contacts involving the ligand-binding AGFCC'C" β-sheet observed in rat[47] and human[54] sCD2 crystals, again likely due to the high net positive charge of the central region of this surface. The CD48 ligand-binding domain had AGFCC'C" topology and was therefore grossly similar to the corresponding domains of CD2 and CD58. The β-strand positions in CD48 resembled those in CD2 and CD244 (Fig. 2.1I), including the distinctive position of the C" β-strand and short DE loop. However, there was a reduction in the size of the FG loop of CD48 vs that of CD2 (by one residue) and CD58 (by two), and an increase in the CC' loop by, respectively, 4 and 3 residues. The real outlier within the CD2/CD58/CD48/CD244 subset was CD244, which had very long FG and CC' loops, and H-bonding between the A and G β-strands extending the full length of the G strand, rather than for a third or half of the strand only. Automated structure comparisons selected CD4 as the most CD48-like structure followed by CD2, CD58, and B7-1. CD244 was the 25th-most similar.[73]

Mutations preventing CD2 binding formed a contiguous surface on the AGFCC'C" β-sheet consisting of three hydrophobic, two polar, and five charged residues. Although still highly charged, this surface was significantly less charged than that of CD58, to the same extent that this surface was less charged for rat CD2 vs human CD2 (Fig. 2.1E). Also, in marked contrast to CD58, this surface was remarkably flat. Deviations from the least-squares planes for atoms on the d1 AGFCC'C" face were 1.5Å for rat CD48 and 1.6Å for rat CD2, compared with 3.0 and 1.8Å for the human equivalents. The complex of CD2 and CD48 therefore seemed likely to exhibit greater surface complementarity than CD2/CD58 complexes, which could have been expected to confer stronger rather than weaker binding,[60,61] suggesting that the detail of binding was different. Isothermal calorimetric measurements indicated that the free energy of rat CD2 and CD48 binding had small, favorable enthalpic and entropic components.[73] Increasing the ionic strength produced a slight reduction in the enthalpy term balanced by a slight increase in entropy, suggesting, once again, that the net contribution of electrostatic interactions to binding was very limited.

2.2.5.2   What We Learnt

a.   The structure of CD48 joined CD2, CD58, and CD244 in the CD2 subset of the IgSF, while adding a second member to the nominal SLAM subgrouping.[75,76] These domains all had very different sequences, and the structure of CD48 was as distinct from CD2 and CD58 as CD2 differed from CD58. CD48 had the least similarity to CD244, which was curious since their genes were closely linked following an apparent gene duplication event. Overall, CD2 family proteins seemed to be of ancient origin, and attempts at further subdivision of the family seemed to be largely pointless.

b. There was apparently no murine *Cd58* gene, whereas *CD58* genes were present in humans, zebra fish, chickens, and mallard ducks.[73] Murine CD2 appeared, therefore, to have developed secondary specificity for CD48, perhaps explaining why the interaction was so weak.

c. We proposed that CD48 bound multiple ligands because its relatively flat binding surface and more limited electrostatic potential vs, for example, CD58, allowed it to tolerate variation in the binding surfaces of new ligands. We obtained support for this notion by characterizing the interactions of rat CD48 with the rat CD244 orthologue (rat 2B4; Ref. 77), and the 2B4-related protein, 2B4R (Ref. 78). Remarkably, although 2B4 and 2B4R had similar affinities for CD48, 15/21 of the residues distinguishing the two ligands aligned with residues forming the CD48-binding, d1 AGFCC'C" β-sheet of rat CD2 (used as an initial structural model of 2B4). This emphasized the rate at which these types of proteins were capable of diverging (EJ Evans and SJD, unpublished). A model of the complex of rat CD2 and CD48 (Ref. 73) required a 7-degree rotation and ~3Å translation of CD48 d1 relative to the position of CD58 d1. It would seem, therefore, that recognition by CD2-related proteins might be permissive of significant levels of topological variation in complex formation.

d. Thermodynamic analysis revealed that the binding of human and rat CD2 to their ligands was substantially different. The rat interaction had approximately equally favorable enthalpic and entropic components.[73] In contrast, a substantially higher enthalpy overcomes a larger, unfavorable entropic barrier for human CD2 binding to CD58 (Ref. 74). The unfavorable entropy in the latter case may have resulted from the loss of flexibility of their binding faces in the complex,[79] and from the ordering of solvent molecules between the poorly matched binding surfaces. The enthalpy of binding of rat CD2 to CD48 was about 25% that of human CD2 binding to CD58 ($-3.5\,\text{kcal}\,\text{M}^{-1}$ compared to $-12\,\text{kcal}\,\text{M}^{-1}$), and much smaller than that for antibody/antigen complexes forming interfaces of comparable area (-6 to $-31\,\text{kcal}\,\text{M}^{-1}$),[80] suggesting that the very flat binding surfaces of the rat proteins were unable to form extensive van der Waals contacts in the complex.[73] The low entropy of binding, on the other hand, might have reflected lower conformational flexibility for these proteins.

2.3 CELL-CELL RECOGNITION AND COSTIMULATION: CD28 FAMILY PROTEINS

CD28-related proteins consist of a set of small, mostly T-cell expressed receptors that bind related small cross-reactive ligands (reviewed in Refs. 81,82). CD28 and CTLA-4 each bind to B7-1 (CD80) and B7-2 (CD86) expressed on antigen presenting cells (APCs), forming a network of interactions. Altering these interactions had been shown to have profound effects on immune responses in disease models. Enhanced antitumor immune responses resulted from transfecting

B7-1 into tumors[83,84] or from using antibodies to block CTLA-4 interactions with B7-1 and B7-2 (Ref. 85). Conversely, inhibition of B7/CD28 interactions resulted in general immunosuppression,[86] reduced autoantibody production,[87] and enhanced skin and cardiac allograft survival.[88] The expression of B7-1, B7-2, CD28, and CTLA-4 is tightly regulated. There are significant differences in levels and timescales, with CD28 in most resting human T-cells being constitutively expressed, whereas B7-2 requires immune activation, whereupon it is rapidly induced on APCs. In contrast, up to 24–48 h is required for B7-1 and CTLA-4 expression after activation.[89]

Without coincident signaling by CD28, which amplifies the transcriptional effects of TCR triggering rather than initiating a distinct gene expression program,[90,91] naive T-cells become anergic when only their TCRs are triggered (reviewed in Refs. 81,92). CTLA-4, in contrast, is a potent inhibitor of T-cell activation.[93] Neither CD28 nor CTLA-4 have any intrinsic catalytic activity and are instead phosphorylated on cytoplasmic tyrosine residues by extrinsic kinases, such as the Src kinase Lck.[94–96] Phosphorylation of CD28 results in the recruitment of PI3-kinase, propagating activatory signaling.[97,98] Antibodies that bind CD28 are either costimulatory (i.e., require additional weak signaling by the TCR) or superagonistic (i.e., active in the absence of TCR triggering).[99,100] The downstream signaling consequences of ligand binding by CTLA-4 are less clear-cut. Phosphorylation could stabilize CTLA-4 expression at the cell surface by preventing internalization via clathrin-coated pits, allowing it to compete for CD28 ligands, reducing signaling,[94,95,101] or bind the phosphatase SHP-2 (Refs. 102,103), although this has been controversial.[82] How phosphorylation of CTLA-4 is "triggered" by ligand binding, however, was completely unknown although it was broadly anticipated to involve receptor conformational changes or oligomerization.[82]

Both in mice and humans, the gene pairs encoding CTLA-4 and CD28, and B7-1 and B7-2, are each closely linked on separate chromosomes,[104,105] which, along with their equivalent domain organization and sequence homology, suggest a history of gene duplication. The CTLA-4 and CD28 ECDs are covalent homodimers of single V-set IgSF domains. B7-1 and B7-2 consist of single V-set and C1-set IgSF domains (reviewed in Ref. 82). CTLA-4 binds bivalently to B7-1 and B7-2 (Refs. 106,107), but CD28 is monovalent.[108] In SPR-based assays, B7-1 binds CD28 and CTLA-4 more strongly than B7-2 does, although relative to its CTLA-4-binding affinity, B7-2 binds CD28 more strongly than B7-1 (Ref. 108), implying on balance that B7-2 is the more activating ligand. CD28 is a poor adhesion molecule[109] even though its affinity for its ligands is comparable to those of conventional adhesion molecules,[110] consistent with costimulatory interactions relying on synapse formation following initial TCR stimulation. Simulations have confirmed that the amount of each complex formed is likely determined by the timing of expression, the affinity and stoichiometry of binding, and by competition for ligands.[111]

2.3.1 sB7-1 (2000)

Work on B7-1 produced the first structure of a costimulatory ligand, revealing unsuspected complexities in the evolution of IgSF signaling and adhesive proteins.[112] The structure suggested reasons why CD28 and B7-1 or B7-2 are poor adhesion proteins despite the reasonably high affinities of their interactions and suggested that stoichiometric effects would have a large bearing on signaling outcomes in T cells.

2.3.1.1 The Structure

Histidine-tagged, selenomethionine-labeled sB7-1 produced in Lec3.2.8.1 cells in the presence of NB-DNJ could be readily deglycosylated[22] and then formed crystals diffracting to 3 Å resolution at a synchrotron source. The crystals belonged to space group $I4_122$ and had cell dimensions $a = b = 57.3$ Å, $c = 298.9$ Å. The structure was determined using multiple-wavelength anomalous dispersion. sB7-1 monomers were slender proteins with dimensions of $23 \times 30 \times 90$ Å^3 (Fig. 2.2A). The two anti-parallel β-sandwich IgSF domains were joined by a short linker resembling that first seen in the ECD of rat CD2; however, the relative domain orientations of B7-1 and CD2 differed significantly.

Domain 1 of B7-1 had V-set topology with β-strands forming DEB and AGFCC′C″ β-sheets. Automated structure comparisons identified d1 of human CD2 and CD4d1d2 as the most similar to B7-1 d1, with the most important defining feature distinguishing them from antigen receptor V-set domains being the lack of twist in the AGFCC′C″ β-sheet. This was due, once again, to B7-1 d1 having its β-bulges positioned immediately after the CC′ and FG turns.[54] Unexpectedly, d2 of B7-1 was more similar to the C1-set domains of antigen receptors and MHC proteins than to d2 of human CD2 or CD4d1d2. The key difference was that d2 of B7-1 had DEBA and GFC β-sheets typical of C1-set domains,[45] that is, with extended D and E β-strands forming the first half of the second β-sheet rather than two short C′ and D strands extending the first β-sheet as in human CD2. The d1 AGFCC′C″ β-sheet of B7-1, identified by mutagenesis as the ligand-binding site, had a similar composition to other sites of protein recognition and therefore substantially fewer charged and more hydrophobic residues than the equivalent region of human or rat CD2, consistent with it binding the more hydrophobic B7-1-binding surfaces of CD28 and CTLA-4, each having at their core the conserved MYPPPY sequence.

The interdomain linkers of B7-1 and human CD2 had identical lengths (7 residues) and remarkably similar main chain conformations, even though only a proline (Pro111) and an isoleucine (Ile113) were conserved in both sequences (B7-1 sequence numbering). However, the positioning of d1 of B7-1 differed from that of CD2 by a 100-degree rotation about the long axis of the molecule and by a 20-degree reduction in tilt relative to the same axis. Along with much longer D and E β-strands of d2, this resulted in the interdomain region of B7-1 burying a significantly larger surface area. The conservation of d2 D and E

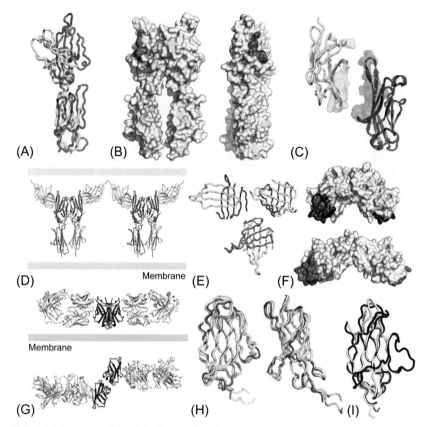

FIG. 2.2   Structures of CD28 family proteins. (A) Schematic α-carbon representations of human sB7-1 (*blue*) and sCD2 (*white*) superimposed on d2 of each molecule. (B) Two orthogonal views of the sB7-1 homodimer observed in the crystals, drawn in surface format and showing the location of residues whose mutation to alanine disrupts binding (*blue*). Putative *N*-glycosylation sites are colored *yellow*. (C) Structures of the interacting surfaces of B7-1 (*blue*) and CTLA-4 (*yellow*) following "undocking" the proteins to a distance of 5–10Å, showing the excellent shape complementarity of the binding surfaces (depicted semitransparently). (D) Molecular association of sB7-1 (*blue*) and sCTLA-4 (*yellow*) in the crystal lattice producing "skewed zipper" arrays. (E) Orthogonal lattice interactions observed in crystals of the sB7-1/sCTLA-4 (*top left*: B7-1 d1 *blue*, CTLA-4 *yellow*) and sCD2/sCD58 (*top right*: CD2 *white*, CD58 *red*) complexes, and in crystals of the homophilic coxsackie and adenovirus receptor (*bottom: orange, white*). (F) Surface representations of the putative CD28 homodimer observed in crystals of the sCD28/5.11A1 Fab complex (*top*) and native sCTLA-4 homodimer (*bottom*). The ligand-binding surface of CTLA-4 is colored *blue* and the structurally equivalent residues in CD28 are colored *dark blue*. Asparagine residues likely to be glycosylated in each protein are *yellow*. In the orientation shown, the C termini (and T-cell surface) are toward the top. (G) Orthogonal views of the complex formed by the putative CD28 homodimer (*dark blue*) and bivalently bound 5.11A1 Fab (*white*). In the top panel, the horizontal *purple* line indicates the approximate position of the membrane with the line of view being parallel with the membrane. In the lower panel, the viewpoint is from above the T cell. (H) The two halves of the apo CTLA-4 homodimer (mol A is colored *yellow*, mol B colored *pale yellow*) are shown superimposed with copies of the CTLA-4 monomer from complexes with B7-1 (*blue*) and B7-2 (*white*). For CTLA-4 complexed with B7-1 and B7-2, the copies shown exhibit the largest differences from mol A of the apo structure. (I) Comparison of the NMR-based (*dark blue*) and crystal (*white*) structures of human sPD-1.

β-strand and DE loop residues forming critical interdomain electrostatic contacts, along with the conserved hydrophobicity of the interdomain core, meant that B7-1 defined a new subset of IgSF proteins with similar topologies, including B7-2, myelin/oligodendrocyte protein, the milk-fat globule membrane protein, butyrophilin, and chicken B-G (MHC) molecules.

A completely unexpected feature of the sB7-1 crystal lattice was the presence of a relatively large contact at the twofold axis burying a total of 1220Å^2 of d1 surface (across both molecules; Fig. 2.2B). This created a compact dimer with similar shape and dimensions to the Fab portions of antibodies except that it involved the interaction of mostly hydrophobic residues in a fairly flat surface formed by d1 B, C″, D, and E β-strand residues rather than the AGFCC′C″ face, and there was no d2 contact. This left the d1 AGFCC′C″ β-sheet free for ligand binding and allowed the C-terminal stalks linking the molecules to the cell surface to enter the membrane adjacently. Ultracentrifugation confirmed that sB7-1 dimerizes in solution with a K_d in the range of 20–50 μM.[112]

2.3.1.2 What We Learnt

a. The topological similarity of d2 of B7-1 to the C1-set domains of antigen receptors and MHC proteins, rather than the C2-set domains of CD2 and CD4d1d2, implied that B7-1-like molecules appeared before the evolution of antigen receptors and MHC proteins. Domain 2 of B7-2, which was clearly related to B7-1, gave equally poor matches to both C1- and C2-set sequences, suggesting it could be even more primitive. The similarity of the adhesion domains of B7-1 and CD2, however, suggested evolutionary relationships in which the earliest C1-set domain-containing proteins were adhesion molecules, and antigen receptors characterized by GFCC′C″ β sheet-mediated V-set domain heterodimerization appeared later.

b. While the B7-1 and CD2 ECDs had similar dimensions, the reduction in the tilt of d1 vs d2 positioned the ligand-binding AGFCC′C″ face of B7-1 nearly parallel to the long axis of the molecule rather than, like CD2, almost normal with it (Refs. 47,54). We proposed[112] that whereas maximum exposure of the ligand-binding face at the "top" of CD2 might be crucial for forming the initial "close-contact" between T cells and APCs,[65] for B7-1, which is expressed following activation, ligand engagement might only be possible after the interacting cell surfaces are optimally aligned. This suggestion was subsequently supported by experiments in bilayers comparing the ability of CD2 and B7-1 to act as adhesion proteins.[109]

c. sB7-1 formed noncovalent homodimers in this and other lattices (SI, unpublished; Ref. 107), and also at the cell surface, as was later shown in resonance energy transfer experiments.[113,114] CD2 seemed to be prevented from forming compact, parallel bivalent homodimers analogous to those formed by B7-1 by the large (42 degrees) tilt in the position of d1 relative to the long axis of the molecule,[47,54] ensuring its monovalence. The K_d of 20–50 μM measured for dimerization of sB7-1 and the rapid monomer-dimer exchange also observed suggested that B7-1 would be in a dynamic equilibrium with monomers, one that was dominated by the homodimer observed in crystal lattices. This was suggested to allow for avidity enhancement of the interaction of B7-1 with CTLA-4, which was already known to have one of the highest affinities (0.2–0.4 µM) described for interacting cell surface molecules (reviewed in Ref. 115). The affinity and stoichiometric differences were calculated to give CD28-family signaling complexes whose stabilities would vary over four orders of magnitude.[108] This implied that an important function of B7-1 was to form particularly stable inhibitory complexes with CTLA-4, late in immune responses.

2.3.2   sCTLA-4/sB7-1 Complex (2001)

The opportunity to consider the structural and functional implications of the crystal structure of the human sCTLA-4/sB7-1 complex arose after Somers and colleagues at Wyeth Research used the sB7-1 crystal structure coordinates (PDB identification number 1DR9) to obtain the phases and solve the structure of the sCTLA-4/sB7-1 complex.[107] Comparisons with ligand binding by CD2 related proteins revealed how particularly stable complexes that suppressed signaling in T-cells were likely formed.

2.3.2.1   The Structure

Fully glycosylated soluble forms of the ECDs of human B7-1 and CTLA-4 were expressed in CHO cells as immunoglobulin Fc fusion proteins by Somers and colleagues.[107] Following removal of the Fc portions proteolytically and mixing at a 1:1.5 molar ratio, crystals belonging to space group $C222_1$ with unit-cell dimensions $a = 88.5$ Å, $b = 183.4$ Å, $c = 230.8$ Å appeared. The structure was solved by molecular replacement. In the lattice, sCTLA-4 and sB7-1 each formed noncrystallographic ~twofold symmetric homodimers. The asymmetric unit comprised single copies of each homodimer.

CTLA-4 and B7-1 monomers did not exhibit any large-scale conformational rearrangements on complex formation. The glycosylated sB7-1 homodimer observed in the complex crystals was essentially identical to that seen previously in the deglycosylated sB7-1 crystals.[112] Although the CTLA-4 monomer was very similar to the murine CTLA-4 monomer solved previously,[116] the homodimers observed in human and murine sCTLA-4 crystals were radically different, suggesting that CTLA-4 might undergo substantial reorganization upon ligand binding. However, formation of the murine CTLA-4 homodimer seemed unlikely: (i) less than half the interacting residues at the murine dimer interface were conserved, (ii) murine CTLA-4 homodimerization was likely to be precluded by glycosylation, and (iii) formation of the dimer would have prevented interchain disulfide bonding.[107] The human CTLA-4 monomers in the complex interacted through mostly hydrophobic A and G β-strand residues, burying 460 Å^2 of surface per monomer. These residues were not conserved in

CD28. Differences noted[116] between the mouse structure and an NMR-derived human sCTLA-4 structure[117] were confirmed in favor of the mouse structure by the complex, including differences in V-set domain topology, and in the *cis* vs *trans* configurations of the prolines forming the [99]MYPPPY[104] sequence of the FG loop.

Complex formation involved the GFCC′ face of the CTLA-4 and B7-1 V-set domains, with an ~90-degree angle between the interacting β-sheets. The FG, BC, and C′C″ loops of CTLA-4 extended across the base of the B7-1 β-sheet burying 1255Å^2 of total solvent-accessible surface, that is, at the low end of the range for protein interactions ($1200–1800 \text{Å}^2$; Ref. 59). Most interatomic contacts were hydrophobic, but there were also five H-bonds. The FG loop of CTLA-4 containing the [99]MYPPPY[104] sequence strictly conserved in CTLA-4 and CD28 dominated binding, contributing 400Å^2 of buried surface. At the core of the interface, Pro102 of CTLA-4 and Tyr31 of B7-1 participated in a stacking interaction likely also to be present in complexes with CD28 and B7-2. Overall, the two binding surfaces exhibited a very high degree of shape complementarity (Fig. 2.2C): measures of the geometric fit between the surfaces[118] gave scores for the CTLA-4/B7-1 complex (0.74–0.77) similar to those for constitutive oligomers (0.7–0.76) and significantly higher than those for interacting cell-surface molecules (0.45–0.58) or even protein antigen/antibody complexes (0.64–0.68). In the crystals, the sCTLA-4 and sB7-1 homodimers formed a periodic array wherein bivalent sCTLA-4 homodimers made orthogonal contacts with bivalent sB7-1 homodimers (Fig. 2.2D).

2.3.2.2 What We Learnt

a. It was known that CTLA-4 formed bivalent homodimers[117] and that the affinity of sB7-1 self-association ($K_d = 20–50 \,\mu\text{M}$) probably ensured that B7-1 is mostly dimeric at the cell surface.[112] Oligomeric arrays of the type observed in the crystals also seemed likely to form at the membrane interface between T cells and APCs. Such an arrangement was reminiscent of the "zippers" observed in cadherin crystals, also thought to mimic interactions in vivo.[119]

b. It was noted that, allowing also for their "stalk" regions attaching the proteins to the membrane, the ECDs of the ligated receptor would span a distance of ~140 Å, similar to that known then to be bridged by TCR/MHC-peptide and CD2/CD58 complexes[51,65,71] and, more recently, by natural killer cell inhibitory receptor/MHC complexes.[120] We have proposed that signaling complexes need to be this small in order that they can be triggered by phosphatase exclusion.[121]

c. Orthogonal interactions involving the GFCC′C″ faces of the V-set IgSF domains of cell-surface molecules were first seen in the sCD2 crystals,[47,54] and later in the native complex of CD2 d1 and CD58 d1 (Ref. 51) and crystals of the coxsackie virus and adenovirus receptor[122] (Fig. 2.2E). There was, and still is, no compelling reason why orthogonal interactions should have arisen convergently, suggesting that these complexes instead bear the imprint of primordial IgSF interactions. We predicted that orthogonal binding would be a recurrent theme of V-set IgSF interactions.

d. The submicromolar affinity of B7-1 for CTLA-4 ($K_d=0.2-0.4\,\mu M$[62]) was unusually high for interacting cell-surface molecules and explained by the relatively high degree of surface complementarity of their interacting surfaces. However, the complex structure further emphasized that potent B7-mediated inhibition relied not only on the strong interactions of individual homodimers but also on the formation of oligomeric arrays of these proteins. Irrespective of the mechanism(s) involved, the inhibition of immune responses by CTLA-4 seemed to require the formation of unusually stable complexes.

2.3.3 sCD28/5.11A1 Antibody Fab (2005)

Work on CD28 was stimulated by its therapeutic potential. However, it was also of interest because we expected the structure to shed more light on interactions at the cell surface generally and among costimulatory proteins specifically. The analysis became of particular interest from a signaling point of view after it became necessary to prepare antibody Fab/sCD28 complexes and we serendipitously obtained a superagonistic (i.e., mitogenic) antibody. Some antibodies were known to be potent agonists of CD28 but not why, although an intriguing correlation was established between epitope location and signaling strength,[123] pointing to a structural explanation; nonmitogenic antibodies bound the ligand-binding region of the V-set IgSF domain of CD28, whereas superagonists bound the C″D loop. The structure of sCD28 monomers bound to the Fab fragment of the mitogenic antibody[124] explained the distinct binding specificities and stoichiometric properties of CD28 and CTLA-4, redefined the evolutionary relationships of CD28-related proteins, antigen receptors, and adhesion molecules, and suggested a new framework for thinking about signaling induced by antibodies.

2.3.3.1 The Structure

Cleaved, fully glycosylated, or deglycosylated sCD28 homodimers expressed as Fc fusion proteins failed to crystallize. Reduction and alkylation gave monomers that produced crystals, but only after mixing with Fab fragments of the mitogenic antibody 5.11A1 (Ref. 123). The crystals diffracted to Bragg spacings of 2.7Å, were of space group $C2$ and had unit cell dimensions of $a=191.2$Å, $b=47.4$Å, $c=71.8$Å ($\beta=94.4$ degrees).[124] The structure was solved by molecular replacement.

The ECD of CD28 comprised an antiparallel β-sandwich of $20\times25\times40$Å^3, with the same DEBA and A′GFCC′C″ β-strand topology as V domains of antigen receptors. Automated structure comparisons showed that, not including CTLA-4, 9 of the 10 most CD28-like domains were V domains, followed then by the V-set IgSF domains of adhesion molecules. The CD28 ligand-binding domain exhibited each of the hallmarks of V domains: (i) substantial β-strand A and B interactions vs the limited A′-G contacts of adhesion molecule V-set domains, (ii) C′and G strand β-bulges characteristic of antigen receptor domains, and (iii) the substantially greater overall twist of the A′GFCC′C″ β-sheet distinguishing V domains from adhesion receptor V-set domains. In CD28, the G strand β-bulge was exaggerated by a side chain/main chain H-bond between the G and F β-strands. In addition, an extended C′C″ loop differentiated CD28 (and CTLA-4) from V domains. As expected, CD28 most resembled CTLA-4, but several differences emphasized their divergence. The exaggerated G strand β-bulge was absent from CTLA-4 and the CC′ loop in CTLA-4 extended beyond the plane of a small, functionally important β-sheet comprising β-strands A′, G′, and F. Also, rather than forming the first strand in the second β-sheet of CTLA-4, β-strand C″ extended the A′GFCC′ face of CD28.

The structure of the FG loop [99]MYPPPY[104] sequence, identified mutationally as the core of the ligand-binding site of CD28 (and CTLA-4), including the *cis-trans-cis* main-chain conformation of the three proline residues, was almost identical in CD28 and CTLA-4.[124] The surface equivalent to that in CTLA-4 buried by B7-1 and B7-2 had very similar contours and electrostatic potential, and exhibited a high degree of electrostatic complementarity with the regions of B7-1 and B7-2 bound by CTLA-4, invoking similar binding modes. Outside this region, the ligand-binding surfaces of CD28 and CTLA-4 defined by the sCTLA-4/ligand complex structures[106,107] were different, explaining the affinity differences for the interactions of each receptor. 5.11A1 Fab bound residues in the C, C′, C″, and F β-strands, and C″D and FG loops of CD28, consistent with mapping data.[123]

The most important lattice contact in the crystals, located at a twofold axis between adjacent sCD28 monomers, seemed likely to mimic native CD28 homodimerization. The contact buried a larger area consisting of residues ideally suited to forming dimer interfaces than the equivalent interface in CTLA-4, but formed a "dimer" with similar shape and dimensions to the CTLA-4 homodimer (Fig. 2.2F). The shapes were similar because dimerization involved residues in β-strands A and G in each case, but otherwise the dimers were fundamentally different. Whereas CTLA-4 dimerization involved residues adjacent to and including the stalk-like region, the putative CD28 dimerization site was formed by a small, three-stranded A′G′F β-sheet present in all IgSF V-set domains. CD28-like homodimerization was prevented in CTLA-4 by the intrusion of the longer CC′ loop into the plane formed by this β-sheet, whereas CD28 avoided CTLA-4-like dimerization owing to substitutions of two hydrophobic residues in the CTLA-4 dimerization site by lysine. Formation of the dimer in vivo would have positioned the Fab portions of CD28-bound 5.11A1 antibody with their long axes roughly parallel with the cell surface (Fig. 2.2G).

Docking B7-1 on the proposed CD28 homodimer guided by the sCTLA-4/sB7-1 complex structure[107] suggested that, rather than being coligated around axes orthogonal to the membrane, the two B7-1 molecules converged, "clash-ing" in the region of d2. This explained why, in binding assays, CTLA-4 is bivalent, whereas CD28 is monovalent.[108] The modeling-based prediction was confirmed by showing that CD28 bound bivalently to B7-1 d1 (Ref. 124). Other evidence that native CD28 formed dimers similar or identical to those seen in the crystals was obtained using cryo electron microscopy-based analysis of a CD28 Fc fusion protein complexed with superagonistic and nonmitogenic anti-bodies. In a third approach, mutations of two residues in the region of the lattice contact were shown to completely abrogate CD28 expression, whereas alter-ing residues that would have formed a CTLA-4-like dimer was well tolerated. Overall, these experiments constituted strong evidence that native CD28 forms homodimers similar to those observed in the crystals, rather than CTLA-4-like homodimers. Finally, the cryo-EM analysis showed that the nonmitogenic an-tibody formed bivalent, V-shaped complexes with the CD28 Fc fusion protein. This confirmed that, like 5.11A1, the non-superagonistic antibody was capable of cross-linking CD28, but formed ~75 Å less-compact complexes (measured along an axis orthogonal to the membrane).

2.3.3.2   What We Learnt

a. Differences in loop and β-strand configuration outside the ligand-binding regions of CD28 and CTLA-4 were consistent with a very ancient dupli-cation of a shared precursor gene. The cores of each ligand-binding site, especially the conformation of the MYPPPY motifs, were nonetheless very similar, explaining why interactions between CD28 and B7 family proteins are detectable across species barriers, for example, humans and chickens.[125] Structural similarities between antigen receptors and CD28 implied that CD28-related proteins and the antigen receptors evolved from a shared an-cestor distinct from conventional adhesion molecules.

b. A key functional distinction between CD28 and CTLA-4 was that CD28 is monovalent rather than bivalent, reducing the stability of signaling complexes formed by CD28 ~100-fold vs those formed by CTLA-4. The structural and binding data revealed that CD28 monovalence results sim-ply from steric interference with ligand binding. Overall, CD28 seemed more likely to exist as stable homodimers like those observed in the lattice than in, as had been proposed, two distinct, that is, "relaxed" and "parallel" conformations.[126]

c. New constraints were also placed on models of antibody-induced recep-tor triggering. CD28 was bivalent for, and would therefore be cross-linked by, both mitogenic and nonmitogenic antibodies. Alongside the finding that CD28 antibodies are not usually mitogenic in solution[123] where cross-linking would be enhanced, these observations suggested that CD28 was not triggered by antibody cross-linking alone. Since antibody-induced confor-mational changes were also unlikely to induce receptor triggering because the structural rearrangements accompanying antibody binding to protein antigens are minimal,[127] it was proposed that antibodies would initiate signaling either by altering the organization of preexisting multicomponent signaling complexes or by effecting the local, size-dependent reorganization of signaling molecules.

2.3.4 sCTLA-4 (2011)

The unusual situation arose that crystal structures of ligand-bound but not apo-forms of human sCTLA-4 had been published, even though two groups had reported obtaining crystals of apo-sCTLA-4 (Refs. 106,128). We had observed[129] that monomers of apo-sCTLA-4 expressed in bacteria according to one of these methods[128] formed β-strand exchanged dimers during crystallization, suggesting that we ought to instead express the homodimer in mammalian cells. The structure of the apo-sCTLA-4 homodimer[130] gave new insights into the mechanism of recognition of CTLA-4 by B7-1 and B7-2, and a deeper understanding of how the CD28-family proteins and antigen receptors had evolved. This work also placed new constraints on how signaling was initiated by this type of receptor. Previously, the only apo sCTLA-4 structure solved was that of the murine homodimer,[116] which was radically different from complexed sCTLA-4 homodimers,[106,107] implying that triggering of the receptor could be dependent on large structural rearrangements.

2.3.4.1 The Structure

The apo-sCTLA-4 homodimer was expressed as a thrombin-cleavable Fc fusion protein in CHO cells in the presence of kifunensine.[23] Following deglycosylation, the homodimer yielded crystals diffracting to Bragg spacings of 1.8 Å, with unit cell dimensions of $a = 43.86$ Å, $b = 51.46$ Å, and $c = 102.85$ Å, and the space group $P2_12_12_1$ (Ref. 130). The structure was solved by molecular replacement. The asymmetric unit comprised a disulfide-bonded homodimer allowing comparisons with the sCTLA-4/sB7-1 and sCTLA-4/sB7-2 complexes, and with sCTLA-4 bound to an engineered lipocalin.[131]

The two monomers in the asymmetric unit were comprised of β-sandwich domains with AGFCC′ and ABED topology as anticipated by Metzler et al.[132] A short eight-residue "stalk" disulfide-bonded at Cys122 linked the IgSF domains to the membrane. Unexpectedly, the two halves of the apo-CTLA-4 homodimer were less similar to one another than to their complexed counterparts, emphasizing that binding is not accompanied by large-scale structural rearrangements (Fig. 2.2H). Automated structure comparisons identified CD28 and PD-1 as the structures most similar to CTLA-4. Important differences between CTLA-4 and CD28 were: (i) the presence of a kink in β-strand G of CD28, (ii) changes in loop-size including extended AB, BC, and CC′ loops in CTLA-4 and a truncated C″D loop, and (iii) H-bonding of the C′ and C″ β-strands resulting from repositioning of the C′C″ loop in CD28. Of key importance was the largely identical conformation of the FG loop [99]MYPPPY[104] sequence forming the core of their ligand-binding surfaces. Only a single water molecule could be found in the unusually dry ligand-binding surface of apo-CTLA-4, whereas 228 waters were detected elsewhere.

After CD28 and PD-1, the next most similar structures to the CTLA-4 V-set domain were 215 antibody or TCR V-domains, differing mostly in loop lengths only. The r.m.s. difference for superposition of CTLA-4 with the most similar TCR Vα domain was 2.09 Å for 102 residues, contrasting with 2.89 Å for 86 residues for the superposition with d1 of CD2. Important shared features with the Vα domain included the long CC' loop and conserved β-bulges in the C' and G β-strands imposing a pronounced twist on the AGFCC' β-sheet. Especially noteworthy was the high degree of sequence conservation and Cα conformation near the G strand β-bulge, that is, GNGTQIYV (CTLA-4) and GDGTQLVV (Vα). In CD2 and CTLA-4, the loops were similar, and the domains differed insofar as: (i) in CD2 there was no H-bonding of the βA and βB strands, (ii) there was no twist of the A'GFCC' β-sheet in CD2 due to repositioning of the β-bulges, (iii) the position of the C" β-strand in CD2 but not CTLA-4 allowed canonical H-bonding and extension of the AGFCC'C" β-sheet, and (iv) CTLA-4 lacked the twist in the FG loop present in CD2 (and also, e.g., B7-1). The analysis of fifty-two V-set IgSF domains using a sequential structure alignment program[133] indicated that the CD28/CTLA-4 family comprises a subgroup of V-set domains distinct from the groupings of CD8, antigen receptors, and "adhesion" molecules, for example, B7-1 and CD2. Overall, there was greater similarity of the CD28/CTLA-4 subgroup to the antigen receptor family, compared to the adhesion set. The analysis suggested that CD28/CTLA-4 family proteins and antigen receptors shared a common ancestor possibly similar to PD-1, with the two families diverging early.

Apo-CTLA-4 comprised a homodimer with its subunits adopting an arrangement favoring orthogonal bivalent interactions with ligands positioned on apposing cell surfaces. Comparisons with the CTLA-4 monomer pairs in the B7-1 and B7-2 complexes[106,107] and the monomer in the lipocalin complex[131] revealed very limited rotational flexibility at the homodimer interface and remarkably few, if any, changes attributable to ligand binding. The only differences were apparent in the B7-2 complex, with slight repositioning of the BC and CC' loops, and of the C" β-strand and neighboring loops, and conformational differences in the G β-strand at its C-terminus. These local variations were distant from the ligand-binding site of CTLA-4 and for no case did the apo monomers differ systematically from all five complexed CTLA-4 monomers. The main chain atom positions of the [99]MYPPPY[104] sequence were essentially identical.

The structures of the complexes formed by CTLA-4 with B7-1 and B7-2, which had not previously been compared, were quite different.[130] Substitution in B7-2, of Val28 vs Arg29 in B7-1, formed a binding pocket in B7-2 that was only filled in part by CTLA-4. This ensured that the B7-1/CTLA-4 complex exhibited better shape complementarity than the B7-2/CTLA-4 complex. Compensating slightly for this, the surface area buried in B7-2 by CTLA-4 was somewhat larger than that for B7-1. Overall, B7-1 bound CTLA-4 in an even more rigid body-like manner than CTLA-4 engaged B7-1. B7-2 binding by CTLA-4 was, however, more complex and bore the hallmark of "induced fit." In CTLA-4 bound- vs apo-B7-2, there was a 2.3–3.5 Å shift of the B7-2 FG loop toward CTLA-4, that was initiated by a ~120 degrees rotation of Phe31 of B7-2 (Ref. 130). This produced a stacking interaction of Phe31 with Pro102 of the ^{99}MYPPPY^{104} sequence of CTLA-4.

2.3.4.2 What We Learnt

a. Ligand binding hardly altered the structure of the CTLA-4 monomer. Remarkably, the structural differences between the ligand-bound and -unbound receptor were, in fact, fewer than those between the two parts of the *apo* homodimer. This strongly implies that CTLA-4 engagement of ligands is rigid body like. At least in part, in contrast, B7-2 binding involved an induced fit.

b. These remarkable similarities between the liganded and apo forms of CTLA-4 strongly supported the notion that significant rearrangements of their ECDs are not a substantial or universal part of the signaling mechanism of this class of receptors.

c. The CD28/CTLA-4 family comprised a subgroup of V-set domains distinct from both antigen receptors and adhesion molecule-related proteins such as CD2, CD4, and B7-1. It is likely that the family precursor for CD28/CTLA-4 diverged at a very early stage from the lineage that produced antigen receptors. This conclusion is based on CD28 and CTLA-4 being intermediate in their divergence from adhesion molecules vs antigen receptors. The distinctive mode of binding focusing on the proline-rich FG loop still conserved in CTLA-4 and CD28 may have allowed rapid divergence elsewhere in the domain. The reliance of CTLA-4 and CD28 on tyrosine phosphorylation by extrinsic kinases, a property shared with antigen receptors, implied that the common ancestor of all these molecules was a signaling protein.

2.3.5 sPD-1 (2013)

PD-1 (programmed cell death 1) has emerged in the past decade as a pivotal molecule in the immune system, especially with regard to its potential as a therapeutic target. Its inhibitory activity was revealed when PD-1-deficient mice were observed to develop strain-specific autoimmunity: sporadic glomerulonephritis on a C57BL/6 background[134] and cardiomyopathy in BALB/c mice.[135] We were among those who showed that *PDCD1* gene polymorphisms in humans confer susceptibility to systemic lupus erythematosus, atopy, and rheumatoid arthritis.[136–138] PD-1 then became a focus of great interest in two stages: first, when it was shown to be responsible for the "exhausted" phenotype of antigen-specific T cells in animal models of chronic infection[139,140] and in human immunodeficiency,[141] and second, when antibodies blocking the interactions of PD-1 with its ligands produced strong antitumor responses in melanoma patients (reviewed in Refs. 2,142).

PD-1 expression is induced upon the activation of T cells, B cells, natural killer cells, and monocytes.[143] PD-1 binds two different B7-family ligands, PD-L1 and PD-L2 (Refs. 144–147). PD-L1 is constitutively and inducibly expressed by T and B cells, dendritic cells (DCs), and macrophages and also on nonhematopoietic cells, whereas PD-L2 expression is upregulated on DCs, macrophages, and mast cells only.[143] PD-1 is proposed to inhibit signaling, in T cells at least, by recruiting the phosphatase SHP-2 to TCR microclusters during immunological synapse formation, blocking TCR signaling.[148] PD-1 is monomeric and consists of a single V-set IgSF domain attached to a transmembrane domain, and it has a cytoplasmic domain with two tyrosine-based signaling motifs.

Despite its immunotherapeutic importance, there had been no published structures of ligand-bound or -unbound forms of human sPD-1, and only the interactions of bivalent forms of PD-1 with its ligands had been studied (reviewed in Ref. 143), and so the true affinities were unknown. We had early access to the structure of a soluble form of human sPD-1 solved by Carr and colleagues (University of Leicester, UK), along with their NMR-based analysis of its interactions with soluble forms of human PD-L1 and PD-L2 that we supplied. Together with detailed affinity and thermodynamic analyses, the structure broadened our understanding of the structural basis of potent inhibitory signaling in lymphocytes.[149]

2.3.5.1   The Structure and Interactions

The ECD of human PD-1 was expressed in a $^{13}C/^{15}N$-labeled form in inclusion bodies in E. coli, and refolded by rapid dilution.[149] Sequence-specific backbone and side-chain resonance assignments were obtained in triple resonance experiments, allowing automated assignment of the NOEs. Fifty-two satisfactorily converged sPD-1 structures were obtained from 100 random starting conformations using 1879 NMR-derived structural constraints.

The structure analysis confirmed that the ECD of human PD-1 consisted of a two-layer β-sandwich with the GFCC′ and ABED β-sheet topology of IgSF domains. Complementing our analysis of CTLA-4 (Ref. 130), automated structure comparisons identified antigen receptor V domains and the V-set domain of CTLA-4 as the structures most similar to the ECD of human PD-1. The only significant difference between human PD-1 and these receptors was the extra flexibility in the region flanked by the C′ and D β-strands. Human PD-1 differed from mouse PD-1 considerably insofar as the BC loop was not stabilized by disulfide bonding to β-strand F, but the most important difference was at the edge of the GFCC′/GFCC′C″ β-sheets where, for human PD-1, β-strand C″ was completely absent (Fig. 2.2I). Substitution of Cys for Pro at position 63 of human PD-1 shortened the C′ β-strand by one residue, redirecting the next eight residues away from strand C′, producing a highly flexible loop. Perturbations of sPD-1 backbone NMR signals induced by sPD-L1 were highly localized to a patch of residues on one face of human PD-1 centered on Gln55 and including β-strand C, C′, E, F, and G residues, along with residues in the BC, CC′, C′D, and FG loops. These residues presumably formed part of an interaction surface, first identified in crystals of mouse sPD-1 and human sPD-L1 (Ref. 150). The sPD-L2 binding was also centered on Gln55 but with fewer contributions from the BC and FG loops. No conformational changes were induced beyond these regions by either ligand.

SPR-based analysis gave K_d values of 8.2 μM and 2.3 μM for human PD-1 binding to human PD-L1 and PD-L2, respectively. The binding of human B7-1 to human PD-L1 ($K_d \sim 19$ μM) was very significantly weaker than had been reported (~1.7 μM).[151] Kinetic analysis revealed that all affinity differences were almost entirely attributable to off-rate variation. The murine interactions were considerably weaker than the analogous human interactions and, interestingly, not substantially different from one another (K_d 30 and 39 μM for mouse PD-1 binding to mouse PD-L1 and PD-L2, respectively). The affinity of mouse B7-1 for mouse PD-L1 was very low ($K_d \sim 80$ μM). Thermodynamic parameterization revealed that human PD-1/PD-L1 binding was entropically driven, whereas the human PD-1/PD-L2 interaction had a large enthalpic term. The lack of effects of temperature, pH, and salt on binding suggested that the differences in affinity and thermodynamic parameters resulted from minor changes in the formation of noncovalent interactions in the binding sites. Finally, complex formation was simulated using a system of nonlinear ordinary differential equations, incorporating stoichiometric, affinity, and expression data. Although human PD-1 bound PD-L2 with a ~3.5-fold higher affinity than it bound PD-L1, PD-L1 dominated the steady state due to the much lower expression of PD-L2 vs PD-L1 (Ref. 149).

2.3.5.2   What We Learnt

a.   The structure of the human PD-1 ECD was most similar to that of antigen receptor V domains, consistent with a shared evolutionary origin.[130] Human PD-1 was surprisingly different from mouse PD-1, however, in that it lacked "conventional" IgSF V-set domain topology insofar as the C′ and D β-strands were connected by a long, flexible loop rather than a C″ strand. Also, the BC loop was not stabilized by a disulfide as in the mouse structure. These receptor differences explained the surprising differences in the human and mouse PD-1 ligand-binding affinities because mouse PD-L1 and PD-L2 had the same affinities for human PD-1 as the human ligands (X Cheng and SJD, unpublished).

b.   The interactions of PD-1 were relatively weak and much weaker than those of the other key inhibitory protein expressed by T cells, that is, CTLA-4, owing not only to affinity differences but also stoichiometric effects. Overall, the half-lives of human PD-1/PD-L1 and PD-1/PD-L2 signaling complexes were as much as 1000- to 5000-fold shorter than that of CTLA-4/B7-1 complexes, with the difference being even greater for the murine interactions.

c. The binding properties of mouse PD-L1 and PD-L2 were essentially the same, suggesting that the two ligands are not required to produce differential signals. However, PD-L1 and PD-L2 are not functionally redundant because CD8$^+$ T cells in PD-L1-deficient mice exacerbate damage in an experimental autoimmune model,[152] whereas these cells are less destructive in PD-L2-deficient mice.[153] These effects could not be explained in terms of the binding properties of the two proteins.

2.4 CONCLUDING REMARKS

The first crystal structure of the ECD of a small leukocyte adhesion molecule, rat CD2, identified the important structure-function relationships for proteins of this type.[47] Flexibility in the interdomain region and the location of ligand-binding sites close to the top of adhesion molecules are likely to be general features of their organization that facilitate ligand engagement. The structure of sCD2, which was otherwise rigid, implied that induced conformational changes were unlikely as explanations for the agonistic effects of certain combinations of anti-CD2 antibodies.[29] We would now invoke, in order to explain the signal-enhancing effects of d2-binding antihuman CD2 antibodies, the steric exclusion of phosphatases, which would favor the net phosphorylation of local, ligand-unengaged TCRs.[8,121] The homophilic association observed in the rat sCD2 crystal lattice, recapitulated in human sCD2 crystals,[54] established a new type of adhesive interaction for V-set IgSF domains. The differences between this and standard antibody V-domain dimerization presumably resulted from a switch from the side-by-side intramolecular dimerization mode observed in antibodies to one suitable for intermolecular adhesion between cells, or vice versa.[46] The unique features of the ligand-binding site of rat CD2, exaggerated in human CD2, that is, its relative flatness and the large fraction of charged residues located there, predicted that ligand binding by CD2 involves primarily electrostatic contacts.[47,54] Mutagenesis experiments[50] established, however, that these residues make only minor, if any, contributions to binding strength and are instead the effectors of binding specificity. We proposed[50] that electrostatic complementarity would have special utility at the cell surface by allowing affinity and specificity to be uncoupled, in contrast to high-affinity interactions wherein specificity and affinity each depend on surface-shape complementarity and allow, especially, hydrophobic interactions to contribute to binding.[59] These principles were reinforced by the structures of human and rat CD2 ligands, although the fine details of binding differ for the two species as shown by thermodynamic analyses.[73,74]

The remarkable levels of invention and variability underpinning protein recognition at leukocyte surfaces were emphasized by the structural analysis of costimulatory proteins, however. Whereas maximum exposure of the ligand-binding site at the "top" of CD2 (Refs. 47,54) likely enhances the initial close contact of T cells with APCs, the positioning of the B7-1 ligand-binding surface on the "side" of the molecule might ensure that binding occurs only after the two cell surfaces are optimally aligned at the immunological synapse.[109,112] In this way, topology may influence both the specificity and timing of interactions. The important role of topology was further emphasized by the structure of the CD28 homodimer, for which a slight rotation of the homodimeric interface converts what would have been a bivalent dimer into a monovalent one.[108,124] Comparisons of the liganded and unliganded forms of CTLA-4 showed that ligand binding is, for the most part, rigid body in nature, firmly ruling out conformational changes as the general mechanism of signaling by these types of receptors, a group that includes the TCR and CD28 (Ref. 130). The stronger B7-1/CTLA-4 interaction vs those of CD2 family proteins is explained by the greater surface complementarity of their interacting surfaces, although the binding strength still falls well short of that, for example, of antibodies binding to protein antigens, most likely because the area of contact is smaller.[107] The formation of B7-1 dimers, on the other hand, allows the interactions of B7-1 with its ligands to be avidity enhanced, contributing to the four orders of magnitude variation in the stability of CD28/CTLA-4/B7-1/B7-2 signaling complexes.[108] In contrast to the inhibitory effects of CTLA-4 that seem to require unusually strong binding, complexes formed by PD-1 are as much as 5000-fold shorter-lived in humans and even more than this in mice, implying that inhibitory signaling does not always depend on the formation of stable signaling complexes.[149] The CD2-like orthogonal interactions of B7-1 and CTLA-4 observed in crystals of the complex are very unlikely to have arisen convergently, and comprise instead the last vestige of primordial IgSF interactions.[107] The topological similarity of d1 of B7-1 and the V-set ligand-binding domain of CD2, and of d2 with the C1-set domains of antigen receptors and MHC antigens suggests that the earliest C1-set domain-containing proteins were adhesion molecules, and that the antigen receptors initiating adaptive immune responses likely appeared later.[112] Similarities of PD-1, CD28, and CTLA-4 to antigen receptors suggest that they all shared, as a common ancestor, a signaling protein, one not unlike PD-1 perhaps.[130,149]

But have these insights stood the test of time, and what more was learnt about protein recognition and the constraints placed on signaling at leukocyte surfaces? We conspicuously failed to produce well-diffracting crystals of the complexes formed by the proteins we had studied. Others, however, were successful in producing, most tellingly, heterophilic CD2/CD58 (Ref. 51), 2B4/CD48 (Ref. 154), and PD-1/ligand[150,155,156] complexes, and the homophilic NTB-A complex.[157] In a *tour de force* requiring multiply-mutated forms of CD2d1 and CD58d1, Wang et al. confirmed that the CD2/CD58 interaction is mediated by orthogonally interacting GFCC'C" β-sheets rather than the 60 degrees packing of V domains observed in antibodies, and that binding is dominated by charged-residue interactions.[51] Indeed, Wang et al. identified a complex network of 10 salt bridges and 5 H-bonds at the interface and just 3 hydrophobic residues. They argued that interdigitating charged residues would contribute both specificity and binding energy by neutralizing unfavorable interactions of like-charged residues clustered in each binding site but such effects can only be small because, like the rat homologues, the binding of CD2 and CD58 is largely unaffected by electrostatic screening.[74] An unexpected finding was that conformational changes focused on the C'C″ and FG loops of CD58 allowed four intermolecular salt bridges to form in the complex, which now explains, at least in part, the unfavorable entropy of binding ($4.4 \pm 0.2 \, \text{kcal·mol}^{-1}$; Ref. 74). Main-chain FG and CC′ loop interactions were observed, as expected,[47,54] but only for the CD2 FG loop and CD58 CC′ loop (i.e., the G90 carbonyl of CD2 with the main-chain nitrogen of K34 of CD58; a symmetrical interaction was precluded by shortening of the FG loop of CD58 relative to CD2; Ref. 51). Wang et al. also confirmed that shape complementarity at the interface is at the very poor extreme for protein-protein interactions, limiting affinity. We tested whether the homophilic CD2 lattice contacts were good models of heterophilic CD2/ligand interactions by attempting to predict the structure of the native complex prior to its publication using the human CD2 lattice contact to guide docking of unliganded CD2 and CD58 (Ref. 67). The model and actual complexes were remarkably similar, exhibiting r.m.s. differences of only 1.57Å and 1.66Å for the two copies of the native interaction observed in the crystals (SI and SJD, unpublished). Although complex topology, based on largely orthogonal interactions of V-set domain GFCC′C″ β-sheets located at the "tops" of each molecule, is broadly similar for CD2/CD58, 2B4/CD48, and NTB-A complexes, the 2B4/CD48 complex[154] is more reliant on loop residues and main-chain interactions, and NTB-A homodimerization more dependent on C, C′, C″, and F β-strand to β-strand contacts.[157] In addition, NTB-A and 2B4/CD48 complexes exhibit more surface complementarity than the CD2/CD58 complex, and whereas the 2B4/CD48 interface depends on charge-charge interactions (although less so than CD2/CD58), homophilic NTB-A binding relies on noncharged H-bonding and the interactions of tightly clustered aromatic residues. Finally, the human PD-1/PD-L1 complex offers a second example of the stabilizing effects of a large loop-region conformational rearrangement and more evidence for mixed polar/nonpolar interactions contributing to binding.[156]

The remarkably Fv-like arrangement of ligand-binding V-set domains in PD-1/PD-L1 and PD-1/PD-L2 complexes[150,155,156] offers the strongest evidence yet that an ancient, side-by-side associating dimer switched to forming intermolecular contacts between cells (or vice versa). As Springer has observed,[46] if the homodimer associated orthogonally via a single domain, such a switch will only have required reexpression of one of the chains on apposing cells, and no other changes in the association mode. If this is what happened, work on the complexes suggests that there has been considerable structural drift away from whatever was the source binding event, with the roughly orthogonal footprint perhaps the only primordial element preserved in these interactions. Clearly, it was far more important that these interactions persisted and were weak than how this was achieved. In this sense, we were fortunate to choose the CD2 family and costimulatory proteins, which turn out to offer extreme examples of the binding modes observed at leukocyte cell surfaces. One consistent finding, however, is that the complexes formed by leukocyte receptors, first glimpsed in lattices of sCD2 crystals, have dimensions of ~150Å orthogonal to the membrane, taking into account the stalk regions absent from most structures. It is generally felt that this allows all the complexes to accumulate at immune synapses, allowing in turn their various signaling effects to be integrated.[154,155,157] The important function of CD2, perhaps, is to establish the "gap" between the interacting surfaces, optimizing it for ligand scanning by signaling receptors and/or preventing collapse of the contact.[65] However, we have conjectured that the assembly of small complexes might also ensure that they form in regions of contact from which the relatively large phosphatase CD45 but not kinases is excluded,[8] in this way "triggering" tyrosine phosphorylation and signaling by the receptors.[121] The coexpression of CD45, known formerly as "leukocyte common antigen" owing to its expression in all leukocytes,[158] with small signaling proteins like CD28 or other small proteins like CD2 that facilitate ligand binding by the small signaling proteins, may have fueled the leukocyte-specific expansion of the large set of IgSF-related signaling proteins now known to be among the key executors of leukocyte function.

ACKNOWLEDGMENTS

The authors thank Professors EY Jones and DI Stuart and their colleagues for their profound contributions to these studies, and the members of the authors' laboratories who did most of the work discussed. They are also grateful to Dr. Yuan Lui for help in compiling the figures.

REFERENCES

1. Benjamin RJ, Waldmann H. Induction of tolerance by monoclonal antibody therapy. *Nature* 1986;**320**:449–51.
2. Sharma P, Allison JP. The future of immune checkpoint therapy. *Science* 2015;**348**:56–61.
3. Köhler G, Milstein C. Continuous cultures of fused cells secreting antibody of predefined specificity. *Nature* 1975;**256**:495–7.
4. Williams AF, Galfrè G, Milstein C. Analysis of cell surfaces by xenogeneic myeloma-hybrid antibodies: differentiation antigens of rat lymphocytes. *Cell* 1977;**12**:663–73.
5. Evans EJ, Hene L, Sparks LM, Dong T, Retiere C, Fennelly JA, et al. The T cell surface—how well do we know it? *Immunity* 2003;**19**:213–23.
6. Monks CR, Freiberg BA, Kupfer H, Sciaky N, Kupfer A. Three-dimensional segregation of supramolecular activation clusters in T cells. *Nature* 1998;**395**:82–6.
7. Varma R, Campi G, Yokosuka T, Saito T, Dustin ML. T cell receptor-proximal signals are sustained in peripheral microclusters and terminated in the central supramolecular activation cluster. *Immunity* 2006;**25**:117–27.

8. Chang VT, Fernandes RA, Ganzinger KA, Lee SF, Siebold C, McColl J, et al. Initiation of T cell signalling by CD45 segregation at 'close contacts'. *Nat Immunol* 2016;**17**:574–82.

9. Davies DR, Padlan EA, Segal DM. Three-dimensional structure of immunoglobulins. *Annu Rev Biochem* 1975;**44**:639–67.

10. Amzel LM, Poljak RJ. Three-dimensional structure of immunoglobulins. *Annu Rev Biochem* 1979;**48**:961–97.

11. Colman PM. Structure of antibody-antigen complexes: implications for immune recognition. *Adv Immunol* 1988;**43**:99–132.

12. Davies DR, Padlan EA, Sheriff S. Antibody-antigen complexes. *Annu Rev Biochem* 1990;**59**:439–73.

13. Bjorkman PJ, Saper MA, Samraoui B, Bennett WS, Strominger JL, Wiley DC. Structure of the human class I histocompatibility antigen, HLA-A2. *Nature* 1987;**329**:506–12.

14. Brown JH, Jardetzky TS, Gorga JC, Stern LJ, Urban RG, Strominger JL, et al. Three-dimensional structure of the human class II histocompatibility antigen HLA-DR1. *Nature* 1993;**364**:33–9.

15. Wang JH, Yan YW, Garrett TP, Liu JH, Rodgers DW, Garlick RL, et al. Atomic structure of a fragment of human CD4 containing two immunoglobulin-like domains. *Nature* 1990;**348**:411–8.

16. Ryu SE, Kwong PD, Truneh A, Porter TG, Arthos J, Rosenberg M, et al. Crystal structure of an HIV-binding recombinant fragment of human CD4. *Nature* 1990;**348**:419–26.

17. Leahy DJ, Axel R, Hendrickson WA. Crystal structure of a soluble form of the human T cell coreceptor CD8 at 2.6 A resolution. *Cell* 1992;**68**:1145–62.

18. van der Merwe PA, Barclay AN. Transient intercellular adhesion: the importance of weak protein-protein interactions. *Trends Biochem Sci* 1994;**19**:354–8.

19. Barclay AN, Beyers AD, Birkeland ML, Brown MH, Davis SJ, Somoza C, et al. *The leukocyte antigen factsbook*. 1st ed. London: Academic Press; 1993.

20. Davis SJ, Puklavec MJ, Ashford DA, Harlos K, Jones EY, Stuart DI, et al. Expression of soluble recombinant glycoproteins with predefined glycosylation: application to the crystallization of the T-cell glycoprotein CD2. *Prot Eng* 1993;**6**:229–32.

21. Stanley P. Chinese hamster ovary cell mutants with multiple glycosylation defects for production of glycoproteins with minimal carbohydrate heterogeneity. *Mol Cell Biol* 1989;**9**:377–83.

22. Butters TD, Sparks LM, Harlos K, Ikemizu S, Stuart DI, Jones EY, et al. Additive effects of N-butyldeoxynojirimycin and the Lec3.2.8.1 mutant phenotype on N-glycan processing in Chinese hamster ovary cells: application to glycoprotein crystallisation. *Proteins* 1999;**8**:1696–701.

23. Chang VT, Crispin M, Aricescu AR, Harvey DJ, Nettleship JE, Fennelly JA, et al. Glycoprotein structural genomics: solving the glycosylation problem. *Structure* 2007;**15**:267–73.

24. Davis SJ, Davies EA, Barclay AN, Daenke S, Bodian DL, Jones EY, et al. Ligand binding by the immunoglobulin superfamily recognition molecule CD2 is glycosylation-independent. *J Biol Chem* 1995;**270**:369–75.

25. Engel P, Eck MJ, Terhorst C. The SAP and SLAM families in immune responses and X-linked lymphoproliferative disease. *Nat Rev Immunol* 2003;**3**:813–21.

26. Hünig T. The cell surface molecule recognized by the erythrocyte receptor of T lymphocytes. Identification and partial characterization using a monoclonal antibody. *J Exp Med* 1985;**162**:890–901.

27. Selvaraj P, Plunkett ML, Dustin M, Sanders ME, Shaw S, Springer TA. The T lymphocyte glycoprotein CD2 binds the cell surface ligand LFA-3. *Nature* 1987;**326**:400–3.

28. Kato K, Koyanagi M, Okada H, Takanashi T, Wong YW, Williams AF, et al. CD48 is a counter-receptor for mouse CD2 and is involved in T cell activation. *J Exp Med* 1992;**176**:1241–9.

29. Meuer SC, Hussey RE, Fabbi M, Fox D, Acuto O, Fitzgerald KA, Hodgdon JC, et al. An alternative pathway of T-cell activation: a functional role for the 50 kd T11 sheep erythrocyte receptor protein. *Cell* 1984;**36**:897–906.

30. Spruyt LL, Glennie MJ, Beyers AD, Williams AF. Signal transduction by the CD2 antigen in T cells and natural killer cells: requirement for expression of a functional T cell receptor or binding of antibody Fc to the Fc receptor, Fc gamma RIIIA (CD16). *J Exp Med* 1991;**174**:1407–15.

31. Killeen N, Stuart SG, Littman DR. Development and function of T cells in mice with a disrupted CD2 gene. *EMBO J* 1992;**11**:4329–36.

32. Bachmann MF, Barner M, Kopf M. CD2 sets quantitative thresholds in T cell activation. *J Exp Med* 1999;**190**:1383–92.

33. González-Cabrero J, Wise CJ, Latchman Y, Freeman GJ, Sharpe AH, Reiser H. CD48-deficient mice have a pronounced defect in CD4(+) T cell activation. *Proc Natl Acad Sci U S A* 1999;**96**:1019–23.

34. Brown MH, Boles K, van der Merwe PA, Kumar V, Mathew PA, Barclay AN. 2B4, the natural killer and T cell immunoglobulin superfamily surface protein, is a ligand for CD48. *J Exp Med* 1998;**188**:2083–90.

35. Garni-Wagner BA, Purohit A, Mathew PA, Bennett M, Kumar VA. Novel function-associated molecule related to non-MHC-restricted cytotoxicity mediated by activated natural killer cells and T cells. *J Immunol* 1993;**151**:60–70.

36. Ames JB, Vyas V, Lusin JD, Mariuzza R. NMR structure of the natural killer cell receptor 2B4 (CD244): implications for ligand recognition. *Biochemistry* 2005;**44**:6416–23.

37. Sayos J, Wu C, Morra M, Wang N, Zhang X, Allen D, et al. The X-linked lymphoproliferative-disease gene product SAP regulates signals induced through the co-receptor SLAM. *Nature* 1998;**395**:462–9.

38. Mavaddat N, Mason DW, Atkinson PD, Evans EJ, Gilbert RJ, Stuart DI, et al. Signalling lymphocytic activation molecule (CDw150) is homophilic but self-associates with very low affinity. *J Biol Chem* 2000;**275**:28100–9.

39. Driscoll PC, Cyster JG, Campbell ID, Williams AF. Structure of domain 1 of rat T lymphocyte CD2 antigen. *Nature* 1991;**353**:762–5.

40. Recny MA, Neidhardt EA, Sayre PH, Ciardelli TL, Reinherz EL. Structural and functional characterization of the CD2 immunoadhesion domain. Evidence for inclusion of CD2 in an alpha-beta protein folding class. *J Biol Chem* 1990;**265**:8542–9.

41. Peterson A, Seed B. Monoclonal antibody and ligand binding sites of the T cell erythrocyte receptor (CD2). *Nature* 1987;**329**:842–6.

42. Sayre PH, Hussey RE, Chang HC, Ciardelli TL, Reinherz EL. Structural and binding analysis of a two domain extracellular CD2 molecule. *J Exp Med* 1989;**169**:995–1009.

43. Staunton DE, Fisher RC, LeBeau MM, Lawrence JB, Barton DE, Francke U, et al. Blast-1 possesses a glycosyl-phosphatidylinositol (GPI) membrane anchor, is related to LFA-3 and OX-45, and maps to chromosome 1q21-23. *J Exp Med* 1989;**169**:1087–99.

44. Wong YW, Williams AF, Kingsmore SF, Seldin MF. Structure, expression, and genetic linkage of the mouse BCM1 (OX45 or Blast-1) antigen. Evidence for genetic duplication giving rise to the BCM1 region on mouse chromosome 1 and the CD2/LFA3 region on mouse chromosome 3. *J Exp Med* 1990;**171**:2115–30.

45. Williams AF, Barclay AN. The immunoglobulin superfamily—domains for cell surface recognition. *Annu Rev Immunol* 1988;**6**:381–405.

46. Springer TA. Cell adhesion. A birth certificate for CD2. *Nature* 1991;**353**:704–5.
47. Jones EY, Davis SJ, Williams AF, Harlos K, Stuart DI. Crystal structure at 2.8 A resolution of a soluble form of the cell adhesion molecule CD2. *Nature* 1992;**360**:232–9.
48. Killeen N, Moessner R, Arvieux J, Willis A, Williams AF. The MRC OX-45 antigen of rat leukocytes and endothelium is in a subset of the immunoglobulin superfamily with CD2, LFA-3 and carcinoembryonic antigens. *EMBO J* 1988;**7**:3087–91.
49. Stuart DI, Levine M, Muirhead H, Stammers DK. Crystal structure of cat muscle pyruvate kinase at a resolution of 2.6 A. *J Mol Biol* 1979;**134**:109–42.
50. Davis SJ, Davies EA, Tucknott MG, Jones EY, van der Merwe PA. The role of charged residues mediating low affinity protein-protein recognition at the cell surface by CD2. *Proc Natl Acad Sci U S A* 1998;**95**:5490–4.
51. Wang JH, Smolyar A, Tan K, Liu JH, Kim M, Sun ZY, et al. Structure of a heterophilic adhesion complex between the human CD2 and CD58 (LFA-3) counterreceptors. *Cell* 1999;**97**:791–803.
52. Chothia C, Novotný J, Bruccoleri R, Karplus M. Domain association in immunoglobulin molecules. The packing of variable domains. *J Mol Biol* 1985;**186**:651–63.
53. Tavernor AS, Kydd JH, Bodian DL, Jones EY, Stuart DI, Davis SJ, et al. Expression cloning of an equine T-lymphocyte glycoprotein CD2 cDNA. Structure-based analysis of conserved sequence elements. *Eur J Biochem* 1994;**219**:969–76.
54. Bodian DL, Jones EY, Harlos K, Stuart DI, Davis SJ. Crystal structure of the extracellular region of the human cell adhesion molecule CD2 at 2.5 A resolution. *Structure* 1994;**2**:755–66.
55. Withka JM, Wyss DF, Wagner G, Arulanandam AR, Reinherz EL, Recny MA. Structure of the glycosylated adhesion domain of human T lymphocyte glycoprotein CD2. *Structure* 1993;**1**:69–81.
56. Wyss DF, Withka JM, Knoppers MH, Sterne KA, Recny MA, Wagner G. 1H resonance assignments and secondary structure of the 13.6 kDa glycosylated adhesion domain of human CD2. *Biochemistry* 1993;**32**:10995–1006.
57. Somoza C, Driscoll PC, Cyster JG, Williams AF. Mutational analysis of the CD2/CD58 interaction: the binding site for CD58 lies on one face of the first domain of human CD2. *J Exp Med* 1993;**178**:549–58.
58. Arulanandam AR, Withka JM, Wyss DF, Wagner G, Kister A, Pallai P, Recny MA, Reinherz EL. The CD58 (LFA-3) binding site is a localized and highly charged surface area on the AGFCC'C" face of the human CD2 adhesion domain. *Proc Natl Acad Sci U S A* 1993;**90**:11613–7.
59. Janin J, Chothia C. The structure of protein-protein recognition sites. *J Biol Chem* 1990;**265**:16027–30.
60. van der Merwe PA, Brown MH, Davis SJ, Barclay AN. Affinity and kinetic analysis of the interaction of the cell adhesion molecules rat CD2 and CD48. *EMBO J* 1993;**12**:4945–54.
61. van der Merwe PA, Barclay AN, Mason DW, Davies EA, Morgan BP, Tone M, et al. Human cell-adhesion molecule CD2 binds CD58 (LFA-3) with a very low affinity and an extremely fast dissociation rate but does not bind CD48 or CD59. *Biochemistry* 1994;**33**:10149–60.
62. van der Merwe PA, Bodian DL, Daenke S, Linsley P, Davis SJ. CD80 (B7-1) binds both CD28 and CTLA-4 with a low affinity and very fast kinetics. *J Exp Med* 1997;**185**:393–403.
63. Nicholson MW, Barclay AN, Singer MS, Rosen SD, van der Merwe PA. Affinity and kinetic analysis of L-selectin (CD62L) binding to glycosylation-dependent cell-adhesion molecule-1. *J Biol Chem* 1998;**273**:763–70.
64. McAlister MS, Mott HR, van der Merwe PA, Campbell ID, Davis SJ, Driscoll PC. NMR analysis of interacting soluble forms of the cell-cell recognition molecules CD2 and CD48. *Biochemistry* 1996;**35**:5982–91.

65. van der Merwe PA, McNamee PN, Davies EA, Barclay AN, Davis SJ. Topology of the CD2-CD48 cell-adhesion molecule complex: implications for antigen recognition by T cells. *Curr Biol* 1995;**5**:74–84.

66. Honig B, Nicholls A. Classical electrostatics in biology and chemistry. *Science* 1995;**268**:1144–9.

67. Ikemizu S, Sparks LM, van der Merwe PA, Harlos K, Stuart DI, Jones EY, et al. Crystal structure of the CD2-binding domain of CD58 (lymphocyte function-associated antigen 3) at 1.8-A resolution. *Proc Natl Acad Sci U S A* 1999;**96**:4289–94.

68. Arulanandam AR, Kister A, McGregor MJ, Wyss DF, Wagner G, Reinherz EL. Interaction between human CD2 and CD58 involves the major beta sheet surface of each of their respective adhesion domains. *J Exp Med* 1994;**180**:1861–71.

69. Osborn L, Day ES, Miller GT, Karpusas M, Tizard R, Meuer SC, et al. Amino acid residues required for binding of lymphocyte function-associated antigen 3 (CD58) to its counter-receptor CD2. *J Exp Med* 1995;**181**:429–34.

70. Shapiro L, Doyle JP, Hensley P, Colman DR, Hendrickson WA. Crystal structure of the extracellular domain from P0, the major structural protein of peripheral nerve myelin. *Neuron* 1996;**17**:435–49.

71. Garboczi DN, Ghosh P, Utz U, Fan QR, Biddison WE, Wiley DC. Structure of the complex between human T-cell receptor, viral peptide and HLA-A2. *Nature* 1996;**384**:134–41.

72. Garcia KC, Degano M, Pease LR, Huang M, Peterson PA, Teyton L, et al. Structural basis of plasticity in T cell receptor recognition of a self peptide-MHC antigen. *Science* 1998;**279**:1166–72.

73. Evans EJ, Castro MA, O'Brien R, Kearney A, Walsh H, Sparks LM, et al. Crystal structure and binding properties of the CD2 and CD244 (2B4)-binding protein, CD48. *J Biol Chem* 2006;**281**:29309–20.

74. Kearney A, Avramovic A, Castro MA, Carmo AM, Davis SJ, van der Merwe PA. The contribution of conformational adjustments and long-range electrostatic forces to the CD2/CD58 interaction. *J Biol Chem* 2007;**282**:13160–6.

75. Veillette A, Latour S. The SLAM family of immune-cell receptors. *Curr Opin Immunol* 2003;**15**:277–85.

76. Wang N, Morra M, Wu C, Gullo C, Howie D, Coyle T, et al. CD150 is a member of a family of genes that encode glycoproteins on the surface of hematopoietic cells. *Immunogenetics* 2001;**53**:382–94.

77. Kumaresan PR, Stepp SE, Verrett PC, Chuang SS, Boles KS, Lai WC, et al. Molecular characterization of the rat NK cell receptor 2B4. *Mol Immunol* 2000;**37**:735–44.

78. Kumaresan PR, Stepp SE, Bennett M, Kumar V, Mathew PA. Molecular cloning of transmembrane and soluble forms of a novel rat natural killer cell receptor related to 2B4. *Immunogenetics* 2000;**51**:306–13.

79. Kitao A, Wagner G. A space-time structure determination of human CD2 reveals the CD58-binding mode. *Proc Natl Acad Sci U S A* 2000;**97**:2064–8.

80. Schwarz FP, Tello D, Goldbaum FA, Mariuzza RA, Poljak RJ. Thermodynamics of antigen-antibody binding using specific anti-lysozyme antibodies. *Eur J Biochem* 1995;**228**:388–94.

81. Greenwald RJ, Freeman GJ, Sharpe AH. The B7 family revisited. *Annu Rev Immunol* 2005;**23**:515–48.

82. Teft WA, Kirchhof MG, Madrenas J. A molecular perspective of CTLA-4 function. *Annu Rev Immunol* 2006;**24**:65–97.

83. Chen L, Ashe S, Brady WA, Hellström I, Hellström KE, Ledbetter JA, et al. Costimulation of antitumor immunity by the B7 counterreceptor for the T lymphocyte molecules CD28 and CTLA-4. *Cell* 1992;**71**:1093–102.

84. Townsend SE, Allison JP. Tumor rejection after direct costimulation of CD8+ T cells by B7-transfected melanoma cells. *Science* 1993;**259**:368–70.

85. Leach DR, Krummel MF, Allison JP. Enhancement of antitumor immunity by CTLA-4 blockade. *Science* 1996;**271**:1734–6.

86. Linsley PS, Wallace PM, Johnson J, Gibson MG, Greene JL, Ledbetter JA, et al. Immunosuppression in vivo by a soluble form of the CTLA-4 T cell activation molecule. *Science* 1992;**257**:792–5.

87. Finck BK, Linsley PS, Wofsy D. Treatment of murine lupus with CTLA4Ig. *Science* 1994;**265**:1225–7.

88. Larsen CP, Elwood ET, Alexander DZ, Ritchie SC, Hendrix R, Tucker-Burden C, et al. Long-term acceptance of skin and cardiac allografts after blocking CD40 and CD28 pathways. *Nature* 1996;**381**:434–8.

89. Lenschow DJ, Walunas TL, Bluestone JA. CD28/B7 system of T cell costimulation. *Annu Rev Immunol* 1996;**14**:233–58.

90. Riley JL, Mao M, Kobayashi S, Biery M, Burchard J, Cavet G, et al. Modulation of TCR-induced transcriptional profiles by ligation of CD28, ICOS, and CTLA-4 receptors. *Proc Natl Acad Sci U S A* 2002;**99**:11790–5.

91. Diehn M, Alizadeh AA, Rando OJ, Liu CL, Stankunas K, Botstein D, et al. Genomic expression programs and the integration of the CD28 costimulatory signal in T cell activation. *Proc Natl Acad Sci U S A* 2002;**99**:11796–801.

92. Sansom DM, Walker LS. The role of CD28 and cytotoxic T-lymphocyte antigen-4 (CTLA-4) in regulatory T-cell biology. *Immunol Rev* 2006;**212**:131–48.

93. Waterhouse P, Penninger JM, Timms E, Wakeham A, Shahinian A, Lee KP, et al. Lymphoproliferative disorders with early lethality in mice deficient in Ctla-4. *Science* 1995;**270**:985–8.

94. Bradshaw JD, Lu P, Leytze G, Rodgers J, Schieven GL, Bennett KL, et al. Interaction of the cytoplasmic tail of CTLA-4 (CD152) with a clathrin-associated protein is negatively regulated by tyrosine phosphorylation. *Biochemistry* 1997;**36**:15975–82.

95. Shiratori T, Miyatake S, Ohno H, Nakaseko C, Isono K, Bonifacino JS, et al. Tyrosine phosphorylation controls internalization of CTLA-4 by regulating its interaction with clathrin-associated adaptor complex AP-2. *Immunity* 1997;**6**:583–9.

96. Schneider H, Schwartzberg PL, Rudd CE. Resting lymphocyte kinase (Rlk/Txk) phosphorylates the YVKM motif and regulates PI 3-kinase binding to T-cell antigen CTLA-4. *Biochem Biophys Res Commun* 1998;**252**:14–9.

97. Prasad KV, Cai YC, Raab M, Duckworth B, Cantley L, Shoelson SE, Rudd CE. T-cell antigen CD28 interacts with the lipid kinase phosphatidylinositol 3-kinase by a cytoplasmic Tyr(P)-Met-Xaa-Met motif. *Proc Natl Acad Sci U S A* 1994;**91**:2834–8.

98. Truitt KE, Hicks CM, Imboden JB. Stimulation of CD28 triggers an association between CD28 and phosphatidylinositol 3-kinase in Jurkat T cells. *J Exp Med* 1994;**179**:1071–6.

99. Tacke M, Hanke G, Hanke T, Hünig T. CD28-mediated induction of proliferation in resting T cells in vitro and in vivo without engagement of the T cell receptor: evidence for functionally distinct forms of CD28. *Eur J Immunol* 1997;**27**:239–47.

100. Siefken R, Kurrle R, Schwinzer R. CD28-mediated activation of resting human T cells without costimulation of the CD3/TCR complex. *Cell Immunol* 1997;**176**:59–65.

101. Zhang Y, Allison JP. Interaction of CTLA-4 with AP50, a clathrin-coated pit adaptor protein. *Proc Natl Acad Sci U S A* 1997;**94**:9273–8.

102. Chuang E, Lee KM, Robbins MD, Duerr JM, Alegre ML, Hambor JE, et al. Regulation of cytotoxic T lymphocyte-associated molecule-4 by Src kinases. *J Immunol* 1999;**162**:1270–7.

103. Marengère LE, Waterhouse P, Duncan GS, Mittrücker HW, Feng GS, Mak TW. Regulation of T cell receptor signalling by tyrosine phosphatase SYP association with CTLA-4. *Science* 1996;**272**:1170–3.

104. Lafage-Pochitaloff M, Costello R, Couez D, Simonetti J, Mannoni P, Mawas C, et al. Human CD28 and CTLA-4 Ig superfamily genes are located on chromosome 2 at bands q33-q34. *Immunogenetics* 1990;**31**:198–201.

105. Howard TA, Rochelle JM, Seldin MF. Cd28 and Ctla-4, two related members of the Ig supergene family, are tightly linked on proximal mouse chromosome 1. *Immunogenetics* 1991;**33**:74–6.

106. Schwartz JC, Zhang X, Fedorov AA, Nathenson SG, Almo SC. Structural basis for co-stimulation by the human CTLA-4/B7-2 complex. *Nature* 2001;**410**:604–8.

107. Stamper CC, Zhang Y, Tobin JF, Erbe DV, Ikemizu S, Davis SJ, et al. Crystal structure of the B7-1/CTLA-4 complex that inhibits human immune responses. *Nature* 2001;**410**:608–11.

108. Collins AV, Brodie DW, Gilbert RJ, Iaboni A, Manso-Sancho R, Walse B, et al. The interaction properties of costimulatory molecules revisited. *Immunity* 2002;**17**:201–10.

109. Bromley SK, Iaboni A, Davis SJ, Whitty A, Green JM, Shaw AS, et al. The immunological synapse and CD28-CD80 interactions. *Nat Immunol* 2001;**2**:1159–66.

110. Davis SJ, Ikemizu S, Evans EJ, Fugger L, Bakker TR, van der Merwe PA. The nature of molecular recognition by T cells. *Nat Immunol* 2003;**4**:217–24.

111. Jansson A, Barnes E, Klenerman P, Harlén M, Sørensen P, Davis SJ, et al. A theoretical framework for quantitative analysis of the molecular basis of costimulation. *J Immunol* 2005;**175**:1575–85.

112. Ikemizu S, Gilbert RJ, Fennelly JA, Collins AV, Harlos K, Jones EY, et al. Structure and dimerization of a soluble form of B7-1. *Immunity* 2000;**12**:51–60.

113. Bhatia S, Edidin M, Almo SC, Nathenson SG. Different cell surface oligomeric states of B7-1 and B7-2: implications for signalling. *Proc Natl Acad Sci U S A* 2005;**102**:15569–74.

114. James JR, Oliveira MI, Carmo AM, Iaboni A, Davis SJ. A rigorous experimental framework for detecting protein oligomerization using bioluminescence resonance energy transfer. *Nat Methods* 2006;**3**:1001–6.

115. Davis SJ, Ikemizu S, Wild MK, van der Merwe PA. CD2 and the nature of protein interactions mediating cell-cell recognition. *Immunol Rev* 1998;**163**:217–36.

116. Ostrov DA, Shi W, Schwartz JC, Almo SC, Nathenson SG. Structure of murine CTLA-4 and its role in modulating T cell responsiveness. *Science* 2000;**290**:816–9.

117. Linsley PS, Nadler SG, Bajorath J, Peach R, Leung HT, Rogers J, et al. Binding stoichiometry of the cytotoxic T lymphocyte-associated molecule-4 (CTLA-4). A disulfide-linked homodimer binds two CD86 molecules. *J Biol Chem* 1995;**270**:15417–24.

118. Lawrence MC, Colman PM. Shape complementarity at protein/protein interfaces. *J Mol Biol* 1993;**234**:946–50.

119. Shapiro L, Fannon AM, Kwong PD, Thompson A, Lehmann MS, Grübel G, et al. Structural basis of cell-cell adhesion by cadherins. *Nature* 1995;**374**:327–37.

120. Boyington JC, Motyka SA, Schuck P, Brooks AG, Sun PD. Crystal structure of an NK cell immunoglobulin-like receptor in complex with its class I MHC ligand. *Nature* 2000;**405**:537–43.

121. Davis SJ, van der Merwe PA. The kinetic-segregation model: TCR triggering and beyond. *Nat Immunol* 2006;**7**:803–9.

122. van Raaij MJ, Chouin E, van der Zandt H, Bergelson JM, Cusack S. Dimeric structure of the coxsackievirus and adenovirus receptor D1 domain at 1.7 A resolution. *Structure* 2000;**8**:1147–55.

123. Lühder F, Huang Y, Dennehy KM, Guntermann C, Müller I, Winkler E, et al. Topological requirements and signalling properties of T cell-activating, anti-CD28 antibody superagonists. *J Exp Med* 2003;**197**:955–66.

124. Evans EJ, Esnouf RM, Manso-Sancho R, Gilbert RJ, James JR, Yu C, et al. Crystal structure of a soluble CD28-Fab complex. *Nat Immunol* 2005;**6**:271–9.

125. O'Regan MN, Parsons KR, Tregaskes CA, Young JR. A chicken homologue of the co-stimulating molecule CD80 which binds to mammalian CTLA-4. *Immunogenetics* 1999;**49**:68–71.

126. Margulies DH. CD28, costimulator or agonist receptor? *J Exp Med* 2003;**197**:949–53.

127. Davies DR, Cohen GH. Interactions of protein antigens with antibodies. *Proc Natl Acad Sci U S A* 1996;**93**:7–12.

128. Chang CY, Fenderson WH, Lavoie TB, Peach RJ, Einspahr HM, Sheriff S. Crystallization and preliminary X-ray analysis of CTLA-4 (CD152) membrane-external domain. *Acta Crystallogr D Biol Crystallogr* 2000;**56**:1468–9.

129. Sonnen AF, Yu C, Evans EJ, Stuart DI, Davis SJ, Gilbert RJ. Domain metastability: a molecular basis for immunoglobulin deposition? *J Mol Biol* 2010;**399**:207–13.

130. Yu C, Sonnen AF, George R, Dessailly BH, Stagg LJ, Evans EJ, et al. Rigid-body ligand recognition drives cytotoxic T-lymphocyte antigen 4 (CTLA-4) receptor triggering. *J Biol Chem* 2011;**286**:6685–96.

131. Schönfeld D, Matschiner G, Chatwell L, Trentmann S, Gille H, Hülsmeyer M, et al. An engineered lipocalin specific for CTLA-4 reveals a combining site with structural and conformational features similar to antibodies. *Proc Natl Acad Sci U S A* 2009;**106**:8198–203.

132. Metzler WJ, Bajorath J, Fenderson W, Shaw SY, Constantine KL, Naemura J, et al. Solution structure of human CTLA-4 and delineation of a CD80/CD86 binding site conserved in CD28. *Nat Struct Biol* 1997;**4**:527–31.

133. Orengo CA, Taylor WR. SSAP: sequential structure alignment program for protein structure comparison. *Methods Enzymol* 1996;**266**:617–35.

134. Nishimura H, Nose M, Hiai H, Minato N, Honjo T. Development of lupus-like autoimmune diseases by disruption of the PD-1 gene encoding an ITIM motif-carrying immunoreceptor. *Immunity* 1999;**11**:141–51.

135. Nishimura H, Okazaki T, Tanaka Y, Nakatani K, Hara M, Matsumori A, et al. Autoimmune dilated cardiomyopathy in PD-1 receptor-deficient mice. *Science* 2001;**291**:319–22.

136. Ferreiros-Vidal I, Gomez-Reino JJ, Barros F, Carracedo A, Carreira P, Gonzalez-Escribano F, et al. Association of PDCD1 with susceptibility to systemic lupus erythematosus: evidence of population-specific effects. *Arthritis Rheum* 2004;**50**:2590–7.

137. James ES, Harney S, Wordsworth BP, Cookson WO, Davis SJ, Moffatt MF. PDCD1: a tissue-specific susceptibility locus for inherited inflammatory disorders. *Genes Immun* 2005;**6**:430–7.

138. Kong EK, Prokunina-Olsson L, Wong WH, Lau CS, Chan TM, Alarcón-Riquelme M, et al. A new haplotype of PDCD1 is associated with rheumatoid arthritis in Hong Kong Chinese. *Arthritis Rheum* 2005;**52**:1058–62.

139. Barber DL, Wherry EJ, Masopust D, Zhu B, Allison JP, Sharpe AH, et al. Restoring function in exhausted CD8 T cells during chronic viral infection. *Nature* 2006;**439**:682–7.

140. Petrovas C, Price DA, Mattapallil J, Ambrozak DR, Geldmacher C, Cecchinato V, et al. SIV-specific CD8+ T cells express high levels of PD1 and cytokines but have impaired proliferative capacity in acute and chronic SIVmac251 infection. *Blood* 2007;**110**:928–36.

141. Day CL, Kaufmann DE, Kiepiela P, Brown JA, Moodley ES, Reddy S, et al. PD-1 expression on HIV-specific T cells is associated with T-cell exhaustion and disease progression. *Nature* 2006;**443**:350–4.

142. Page DB, Postow MA, Callahan MK, Allison JP, Wolchok JD. Immune modulation in cancer with antibodies. *Annu Rev Med* 2014;**65**:185–202.

143. Keir ME, Butte MJ, Freeman GJ, Sharpe AH. PD-1 and its ligands in tolerance and immunity. *Annu Rev Immunol* 2008;**26**:677–704.

144. Dong H, Zhu G, Tamada K, Chen L. B7-H1, a third member of the B7 family, co-stimulates T-cell proliferation and interleukin-10 secretion. *Nat Med* 1999;**5**:1365–9.

145. Freeman GJ, Long AJ, Iwai Y, Bourque K, Chernova T, Nishimura H, et al. Engagement of the PD-1 immunoinhibitory receptor by a novel B7 family member leads to negative regulation of lymphocyte activation. *J Exp Med* 2000;**192**:1027–34.

146. Latchman Y, Wood CR, Chernova T, Chaudhary D, Borde M, Chernova I, et al. PD-L2 is a second ligand for PD-1 and inhibits T cell activation. *Nat Immunol* 2001;**2**:261–8.

147. Tseng SY, Otsuji M, Gorski K, Huang X, Slansky JE, Pai SI, et al. B7-DC, a new dendritic cell molecule with potent costimulatory properties for T cells. *J Exp Med* 2001;**193**:839–46.

148. Yokosuka T, Takamatsu M, Kobayashi-Imanishi W, Hashimoto-Tane A, Azuma M, Saito T. Programmed cell death 1 forms negative costimulatory microclusters that directly inhibit T cell receptor signalling by recruiting phosphatase SHP2. *J Exp Med* 2012;**209**:1201–17.

149. Cheng X, Veverka V, Radhakrishnan A, Waters LC, Muskett FW, Morgan SH, et al. Structure and interactions of the human programmed cell death 1 receptor. *J Biol Chem* 2013;**288**:11771–85.

150. Lin DY, Tanaka Y, Iwasaki M, Gittis AG, Su HP, Mikami B, et al. The PD-1/PD-L1 complex resembles the antigen-binding Fv domains of antibodies and T cell receptors. *Proc Natl Acad Sci U S A* 2008;**105**:3011–6.

151. Butte MJ, Peña-Cruz V, Kim MJ, Freeman GJ, Sharpe AH. Interaction of human PD-L1 and B7-1. *Mol Immunol* 2008;**45**:3567–72.

152. Dong H, Zhu G, Tamada K, Flies DB, van Deursen JM, Chen L. B7-H1 determines accumulation and deletion of intrahepatic CD8(+) T lymphocytes. *Immunity* 2004;**20**:327–36.

153. Shin T, Yoshimura K, Shin T, Crafton EB, Tsuchiya H, Housseau F, et al. In vivo costimulatory role of B7-DC in tuning T helper cell 1 and cytotoxic T lymphocyte responses. *J Exp Med* 2005;**201**:1531–41.

154. Velikovsky CA, Deng L, Chlewicki LK, Fernández MM, Kumar V, Mariuzza RA. Structure of natural killer receptor 2B4 bound to CD48 reveals basis for heterophilic recognition in signalling lymphocyte activation molecule family. *Immunity* 2007;**27**:572–84.

155. Lázár-Molnár E, Yan Q, Cao E, Ramagopal U, Nathenson SG, Almo SC. Crystal structure of the complex between programmed death-1 (PD-1) and its ligand PD-L2. *Proc Natl Acad Sci U S A* 2008;**105**:10483–8.

156. Zak KM, Kitel R, Przetocka S, Golik P, Guzik K, Musielak B, et al. Structure of the complex of human Programmed Death 1, PD-1, and its ligand PD-L1. *Structure* 2015;**23**:2341–8.

157. Cao E, Ramagopal UA, Fedorov A, Fedorov E, Yan Q, Lary JW, et al. NTB-A receptor crystal structure: insights into homophilic interactions in the signalling lymphocytic activation molecule receptor family. *Immunity* 2006;**25**:559–70.

158. Fabre JW, Williams AF. Quantitative serological analysis of a rabbit anti-rat lymphocyte serum and preliminary biochemical characterisation of the major antigen recognised. *Transplantation* 1977;**23**:349–59.

Chapter 3

Synthetic Antibody Engineering: Concepts and Applications

Jonathan R. Lai*, Gang Chen[†], Sachdev S. Sidhu[†]
*Albert Einstein College of Medicine, Bronx, NY, United States, [†]University of Toronto, Toronto, ON, Canada

3.1 INTRODUCTION

Monoclonal antibodies (mAbs) are widely used as research, diagnostic, and therapeutic reagents. Historically, mAbs have been isolated from mice via hybridoma technology, a process whereby splenic B-cells of immunized animals are fused with myeloma cells to produce a hybrid cell that secretes the desired antibody and can be readily cultured and propagated.[1] More recently, however, alternative methods for isolating mAbs from de novo designed antibody libraries have become available and widely adopted.[2–6] The design of these libraries utilizes bioinformatic and structural information from existing antibody-antigen complexes, to develop specialized randomization schemes at specific sites on the antibody. The diversity of the library is encoded by designed, synthetic oligonucleotides (synthetic antibodies). Antibody fragments as large as antigen-binding fragment (Fab) dimers have been expressed on phage and can be selected readily against various antigens. Other molecular display formats, such as yeast display and mRNA display, have also been employed for antibody engineering.[7,8] Such approaches have advantages over hybridoma methods in that the starting antibody scaffold can be designated from the beginning, allowing selection of a scaffold with particularly desirable properties such as homology to human antibodies and high structural stability. Furthermore, since the selection process is entirely independent of immunization and hybridoma cell fusion, isolation of mAbs from naïve phage display libraries is not subject to intrinsic biases of immunodominance or capacity of particular clones to fuse readily with myeloma fusion partners. The state of the antigen can be precisely controlled during the antibody library selection process, as opposed to requiring formulation with adjuvants that might denature the antigen and thus eliminate the possibility of conformation-specific antibodies. In this chapter, we discuss structural aspects of antibody

Structural Biology in Immunology. https://doi.org/10.1016/B978-0-12-803369-2.00003-6

recognition and library design and then highlight several examples of such approaches from the literature.

The specific interaction between an antibody combining site and its target antigen underlies the basis of all mAb applications and, as such, the known and predictable specificity of mAb binding is critical for function. Therefore, mAbs provide the advantage over polyclonal antibodies (pAbs) for research and diagnostic uses because a mAb is a single known entity whose exact binding parameters (e.g., affinity) and specificities can be determined with a high degree of confidence. In contrast, pAbs generally consist of fractionated immunoglobulin from immunized animals and are thus heterogeneous. Furthermore, recombinant production of mAbs provides an additional level of quality assurance, since large-scale manufacturing can be controlled and repeated stringently with a high level of reproducibility. pAbs can vary from batch to batch because animals can have different responses to similar immunizations and reproducibility is difficult to control in the context of heterogeneous mixtures. Generation of recombinantly expressed mAbs against new and existing targets is now highly scalable, and thus an appealing approach to providing validated and reproducible mAbs for research is to systematically generate and catalog such reagents in a coordinated effort across multiple teams. An example of such team work has been provided recently by the Recombinant Antibody Network, which consists of groups at three sites that have worked together to generate antibodies against hundreds of human transcription factors.[9]

To date, over 70 mAb products have been FDA approved as therapies for a wide range of indications including oncology, inflammation, and infectious disease. The majority of therapeutic mAbs function by disrupting protein-protein or other interactions in the bloodstream or at the cell surface in order to block or enhance particular signaling pathways. In some cases, the Fc (fragment crystallizable)-related functions of the mAb may also play a role or provide a mechanism for therapeutic activity. Two important considerations for therapeutic mAb development are whether the antibody scaffold is of human origin, or from other species, the latter of which is a concern for antitherapeutic mAb immunogenicity; and the specificity profile of the mAb, since off-target binding may lead to undesirable side effects in vivo. Of the FDA-approved mAb products, 7 were isolated or optimized by phage display.[10] In addition to canonical IgG scaffolds, mAbs can be further engineered to contain chemically conjugated drugs (antibody-drug conjugate) or to exhibit specificity toward multiple antigens simultaneously (e.g., bispecific antibodies).[11,12] Bispecific antibodies are often engineered by grafting two sets of variable domains from two separate mAbs into a single, engineered molecule. Often, the bispecific antibody is designed to bring two different cell types together spacially, and a large number of formats are available for bispecific antibody design.[11]

3.2   IMMUNOGLOBULIN STRUCTURE AND FUNCTION

The canonical IgG1 contains two copies of the light chain (each containing a variable domain, VL, and constant domain, CL), two copies of the heavy chain (variable domain, VH, and three constant domains, CH1, CH2, and CH3), and a hinge region between CH1 and CH2 (Fig. 3.1). The two heavy chains are disulfide bonded to one another via two cysteines in the hinge region, and the light chain and heavy chain are joined by a disulfide bond between CL and CH1. The entire IgG1 assembly (150 kDa) is too large to allow efficient display on bacteriophage and contains glycosylation sites in the Fc segment that cannot be recapitulated in bacterial systems. However, full-length IgGs have been expressed in aglycosylated form in *Escherichia coli* periplasm (sometimes as a covalent attachment to periplasmic proteins), and in glycosylated form in yeast.[13,14] Various fragments have been displayed on phage, including single-chain variable fragments (scFvs), antigen-binding fragments (Fabs), and (Fab)$_2$ dimers that include the hinge region to drive dimerization.

All domains within the IgG including the variable domains adopt a β-sheet Ig fold. The variable domains, positioned at the ends of the arms of the Y-shaped

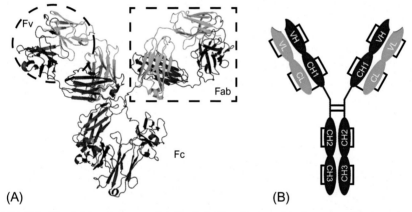

(A)   (B)

FIG. 3.1   The full-length immunoglobulin G (IgG) molecule and its fragments. (A) A cartoon representation of an IgG antibody based on an X-ray crystallographic structure (PDB ID: 1IGY). The IgG molecule comprises two heavy chains and two light chains, shown in *blue* and *green*, respectively, which associate to form a heterodimer with two identical antigen-binding sites at the tip of each antigen-binding fragment (Fab). Six CDRs (shown in *red*), three each from light and heavy chains, collectively form the antigen-binding site that mediates antigen recognition. The dashed box and oval outline two antibody fragments that are commonly used for phage-displayed libraries: the Fab and the Fv. The Fv is typically displayed in the form of a scFv, in which the heavy and light chains are joined together by a polypeptide linker. The Fc is also labeled. Structures were generated by using PyMOL (DeLano Scientific, San Carlos, CA). (B) A schematic representation of the IgG structure color-coded as in A. The subunit composition and domain distribution along the polypeptide chains are shown. Intrachain and interchain disulfide bonds are denoted by a square bracket or a straight line, respectively.

IgG, contain six hypervariable loops (the "complementarity-determining regions" or CDRs) that form the major contact points for most antibodies. Three CDRs are found on each variable domain, heavy and light (CDR-H1, -H2, and -H3 and CDR-L1, -L2, and -L3, respectively). Structural surveys have shown that CDR-H3, which contains the most variation in terms of sequence and length, is the most heavily utilized CDR for antigen binding.[15] In many mAb-antigen interactions, CDR-L3, CDR-H1, and CDR-H2 also play a role, and these segments are targeted for mutagenesis in synthetic antibody libraries. CDRs can be classified according to several canonical loop conformations, with certain positions playing more structural roles and other positions more likely to participate in antibody-antigen interactions.[16]

During natural antibody evolution, a naïve repertoire is generated from recombination of allelic germline segments. For the heavy chain, this includes three regions, the V, D, and J regions. Roughly, the D segment, which is the most variable in terms of length and amino acid sequence, corresponds to the CDR-H3 portion of VH. Naïve light chains are assembled from two segments, V and J, and may be of kappa or lambda origin. Initial diversity is introduced by recombination of the 51 possible V regions, 27 possible D regions, 6 possible J regions; and similarly ~40 Vκ regions, 5 Jκ regions or 122 Vλ regions, and 5 Jλ regions, as well as site-specific mutations introduced by the enzyme activation-induced cytidine deaminase (AID).[17] During antibody responses, the process of affinity maturation and clonal selection drives preferential expansion of higher affinity clones. In the case of antibodies that bind small molecules (haptens), it has been shown that the accumulated somatic hypermutations (SHMs) in some cases improve affinity not by optimizing direct contacts with the hapten, but instead by stabilizing productive CDR loop conformations.[18–20] To this end, the CDR segments of "germline reverted" antibodies are thought to be more flexible, and indeed germline-mimicking antibodies have been shown to be cross-reactive. For protein-binding antibodies, which bear a more extended combining site relative to hapten-targeting mAbs, which contain a well-defined pocket, the SHMs in one case served to optimize the VH-VL interface contacts.[21] Presumably, this mechanism stabilizes productive interactions. For most affinity-matured mAbs, the shape complementarity (Sc) between the antibody and its target appears to be an important correlate of affinity.

While the primary sequences of CDR segments of naïve and matured (i.e., functional) antibodies vary considerably, it is clear that overall there are systematic biases toward certain amino acids.[22] For example, both naive and functional CDR-H3 segments are highly enriched for tyrosine. Functional CDR segments also contain a higher content of serine, glycine, and alanine. Presumably, the physicochemical properties of these side chains are particularly suitable for intermolecular interactions, though tyrosine and serine are also overrepresented in CDR-H3 segments of naïve antibodies, suggesting that there is also some intrinsic bias to the composition of the repertoire toward these residues.[3] Cysteine is underrepresented in functional CDR segments, presumably because unpaired cysteines are a liability for non-native disulfide bond formation, which would compromise structural integrity.

3.3 ENGINEERING PHAGE-DISPLAYED ANTIBODY LIBRARIES

Phage display is an elegant technology whereby the products of gene fragments encoding antibody fragments (either in scFv or Fab format), other proteins or peptides, when fused to filamentous phage coat protein genes within the virus genome or a phagemid vector, can be displayed on the surface of phage particles. In this way, the established physical linkage between phenotype and genotype provides critical complementary sets of information such as function of the protein and sequence of the gene. When phage display was introduced in the mid-1980s,[23] initial efforts were focused on development of peptides with specific binding properties. With advances in the fields of protein engineering and molecular biology, in particular recombinant expression of heterologous complex proteins such as antibody fragments in *E. coli* and PCR technology that allowed for amplification of diverse gene sequences with ease, similar efforts were attempted to identify specific binding proteins from large combinatorial libraries.[24] Since then it has become possible to produce large libraries of antibody fragments in vitro and identify antibodies with desired characteristics by phage selection.[2,25] The coupling of combinatorial library technology and phage selection revolutionized antibody development and was regarded as a major breakthrough in antibody research.

Typically, for generation of mAbs with high affinity from a functional antibody library, monovalent Fab or scFv display through recombinant fusion to the minor coat protein pIII or a fragment of pIII is preferred.[26] The monovalent displayed antibody library undergoes biopanning, a process of multiple rounds of selection on a purified antigen or on antigen-expressing cells, resulting in removal of nonbinding phage and enrichment of antigen-specific phage particles, achieved by amplification of the retained phage pool in an *E. coli* host. In addition, biopanning can be adapted to positively or negatively select desired antibody properties such as affinity, specificity, and stability. Eventually a population that is dominated by antigen-binding clones can be obtained and individual phage clones can be isolated, tested, and subjected to DNA sequencing to decode the sequences of the displayed antibodies (Fig. 3.2).

A functional antibody library of high quality allows for isolation of antibodies against a large collection of diverse antigens with high affinity and specificity. In this regard, natural antibody repertoires have a long-standing proven track record of producing high quality, functional antibodies. Therefore, early approaches for phage displayed antibody library construction relied on capturing diversity of natural repertoires by amplifying VH and VL genes (or their encoded CDRs) from natural genetic sources (i.e., immunized or naïve

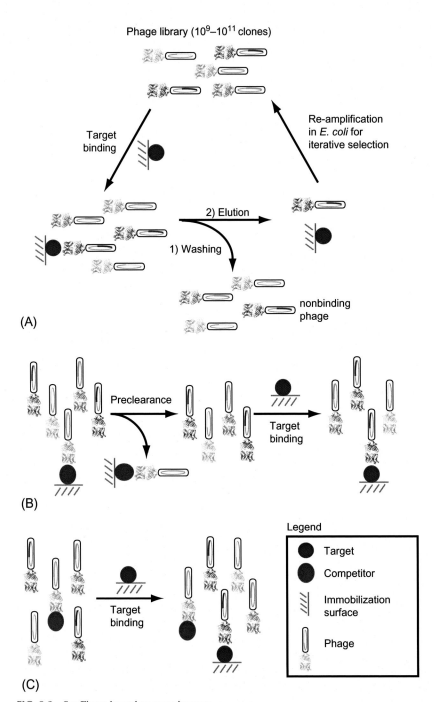

Phage library (10^9–10^{11} clones)

Target binding

Re-amplification in *E. coli* for iterative selection

2) Elution

1) Washing

nonbinding phage

(A)

Preclearance

Target binding

(B)

Target binding

(C)

Legend

● Target

● Competitor

/// Immobilization surface

▯ Phage

FIG. 3.2   See Figure legend on opposite page

B-cells from various tissues or in circulation) followed by grafting them into recombinant display systems for selection in vitro.[2,25,27,28] Construction of these libraries does not require predetermined extensive knowledge of antibody variable domain sequences and only standardized methodology is needed for library generation. Libraries generated in this approach with naïve repertoires were reported to be large and diverse enough to isolate high-affinity antibodies to any given antigen.[28] However, antibody libraries constructed with naïve repertoires often yield antibodies with low affinities and polyreactivity due to the absence of in vivo affinity maturation against the antigen. These mAbs need to be improved by affinity maturation in vitro. More often, natural repertoire-derived antibody libraries are built with immunized B-cell populations with immunity related to certain infections, vaccination, and tumor antigens. This approach provided an efficient means for the enrichment of binding activities already evolved by the natural repertoire.[27,29] These libraries are now still commonly used to generate functional antibodies with clinical potential. However, libraries derived from nonhuman immune repertoires are not suitable for therapeutic application due to potential immune response in humans. mAbs from these libraries must be humanized for potential human use, which is time-consuming and still does not yield fully human antibodies. In comparison, human immune repertoires lack both availability and accessibility although they are highly attractive because they often yield high-affinity mAbs with minimal immunogenicity and off-target reactivity.[30] In addition, libraries derived from natural repertoires randomly combine VH and VL pairs during library generation, which may produce weaker or less stable antibodies compared to original natural sources, while at the same time may yield antibodies with new target recognition beyond the scope of original natural sources.

Unlike antibody libraries built on natural antibody repertoires, antibody libraries with synthetic repertoires have been developed that circumvent the need for a natural repertoire source. These libraries utilize designed synthetic DNA to introduce diversity within antigen-binding sites built in the context of defined

---

FIG. 3.2 Antibody selection by phage display. (A) Highly diverse libraries (10^9–10^{11}) of antibody fragments (Fabs, scFvs, or other autonomous fragments) are displayed on the surfaces of phage particles as fusions to a coat protein. Each phage particle encapsulates a vector containing the DNA encoding a unique antibody, which is displayed on the surface of the same phage particle. In phage selection, the phage libraries are subjected to an iterative process called biopanning where the phage pools are directed in selections for binding to immobilized target, the nonbinding phage are removed by washing, and target-binding phage are retained by the immobilized target and amplified by reinfection of an *E. coli* host. Additional rounds of selection can then ensue. Eventually a population dominated by target-binding phage particles can be obtained. At this stage, individual phage clones can be isolated and subjected to DNA sequencing to decode the sequence of the displayed antibodies. Under certain circumstances, where generation of precise region-specific antibodies is required, a preabsorption treatment before target binding by preclearing the phage pools with immobilized competitor to remove competitor-binding clones (B) can be adopted, or excess competitor can be added into phage pool solution (C) to prevent undesired clones from binding to the target.

frameworks. As the diversity can be introduced at will, one of the evident strengths of synthetic antibody libraries is that diversity similar or alien to natural immune repertoires, or even a combination of both, could be potentially introduced without inherent biases, thus enabling recognition of targets beyond the natural scope.

One strategy to design library diversity is to mimic natural antibody repertoires. Most early synthetic antibody libraries were built through this approach.[31–33] For example, facilitated by in-depth analysis of natural human repertoires and the sequence and length variability of naturally rearranged human antibodies, complex synthetic antibody libraries with $>10^{10}$ independent clones were constructed based on a collection of selected frameworks in which CDR sequences were diversified according to position-dependent occurrence of amino acids in corresponding CDRs in natural repertoires.[33–35] This was achieved by using trinucleotide assembly of mutagenic modular CDR cassettes, a highly tunable process that allows for adaptation of amino acid frequencies in as many as six CDRs as well as length variations in the CDR loops for optimization of various paratope surfaces sampled by the libraries. The fully synthetic nature of library construction also allowed for taking into consideration codon optimization for bacterial and mammalian expression systems, removal of unfavorable residues that promote protein aggregation, and modular gene design to facilitate CDRs accessibility and conversion between different antibody formats.[33] The latest positional amino acid frequency libraries were built on rationally selected VH/VL framework pairs based on desired biophysical characteristics relevant for antibody selection, development, and manufacturing.[36] Library diversity was introduced to remove potential posttranslational modification (PTM) sites. These libraries performed well against various antigens, capable of producing highly diverse sets of unique antibodies with high affinity and high specificity as well as good biophysical characteristics.

Another strategy adopts the spirit of minimalist principles in protein engineering to antibody library design, which led to the generation of fully synthetic antibody libraries. One basic question was raised at the time of this effort: how complex does amino acid composition need to be to create a highly diverse functional paratope set in one or a few selected frameworks that recognize a versatile collection of targets with high affinity and specificity? To address this question, the functional limit of reduced amino acid diversity was put to the test. Initial efforts demonstrated that CDR sequence diversity can be restricted to a quaternary amino acid code (Ala, Asp, Ser, and Tyr)[4] or even a binary code (Ser and Tyr)[3,22] to yield functional antibodies. These minimalist antibody libraries demonstrated the versatility of synthetic repertoires and the capability of precise control over the composition of diversity incorporated in CDRs, and they provided valuable insights into fundamental molecular mechanisms of antibody-antigen recognitions. Moreover, this allowed for systematic optimization of library diversity to achieve a higher level of performance. Over the years minimalist antibody libraries have been progressively optimized and the reduced chemical diversity has also been expanded to balance the minimalist design and library performance.[5,37] The most recent optimized minimalist antibody library was built with limited binary diversity in CDRs H1 and H2 and combinations of nine different amino acids with different weighted matrix in CDRs H3 and L3 (Fig. 3.3). The library was highly functional and allowed for generation of specific Abs that recognized diverse antigens with affinities in the low nanomolar range.[5] Moreover, analysis of antibody clones isolated from this library indicated a significant fraction of antibodies generated against a panel of antigens contained diversified CDR-L3 sequences and a fixed CDR-H3, suggesting that CDR-L3 plays a dominant role in these antibodies, which is contradictory to the classic view that CDR-H3 holds the majority of chemical diversity and naturally plays a dominant role in antigen recognition.[39,40] Therefore, synthetic antibody libraries potentially bear the capacity of developing antibodies from vast combinatorial space, which nature has only sparsely sampled.

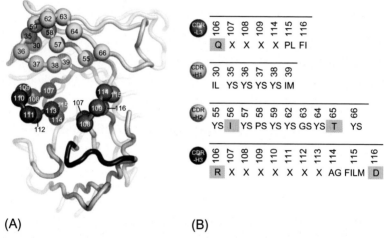

(A)   (B)

FIG. 3.3 Design of a synthetic phage-displayed antibody library. Library F was constructed on a single optimized human framework. Chemical diversity was introduced in all three heavy-chain CDRs and CDR-L3.[5] (A) Close-up view of the antigen-binding site formed by the VL and VH domains (PDB ID: 1FVC). The framework is shown as *gray* tubes. The CDR loops and residue numbering are defined according to the IMGT numbering.[38] Spheres represent positions that were diversified and are colored according to the CDR coloring scheme as follows: CDR-L1, *blue*; CDR-L2, *green*; CDR-L3 *magenta*; CDR-H1, *cyan*; CDR-H2, *yellow*; CDR-H3, *red*. (B) CDR diversity design. Positions fixed as the parental sequence were shaded in *gray*. At each diversified position, the allowed amino acids are denoted by the single-letter code. Single-letter abbreviations for the amino acid residues are as follows: A, Ala; D, Asp; F, Phe; G, Gly; H, His; I, Ile; L, Leu; M, Met; P, Pro; Q, Gln; R, Arg; S, Ser; T, Thr; V, Val; W, Trp; and Y, Tyr. X denotes a mixture of nine amino acids (Y, S, G, A, F, W, H, P, and V) introduced in a ratio of 5:4:4:2:1:1:1:1:1. This was achieved by using a custom trimer phosphoramidite mixture containing nine trimers encoding the aforementioned nine amino acids at defined proportions in the synthesis of the oligonucleotides for library construction. Additional diversity was introduced in the form of multiple lengths of CDR-L3 and -H3; the number of positions denoted by X in CDR-L3 and -H3 varies from 3 to 7 and 1 to 17, respectively (not shown in the figure).

3.4 APPLICATIONS

As discussed earlier, synthetic antibody technology offers an alternative to classic hybridoma technology and enables the rapid development of antibodies through in vitro selections. More importantly, synthetic repertoires make possible precise control of library diversity and antibody frameworks with favorable properties. When combined with precise control of user-specified selection stringency over the evolution process, the synthetic approach offers much broader application scope that is beyond conventional methods, as exemplified by development of antibodies generated to recognize structured RNA molecules,[41] which are nonimmunogenic and essentially impossible to target by classic animal immunization. In vitro antibody technologies also provide various effective means for achieving particular criteria in different applications, such as antibody-assisted crystallization of membrane proteins,[42,43] targeting specific epitopes or viral pathogen intermediates,[44] and development of broad-specificity antibodies against various subtypes of bacterial or viral pathogens.[45,46] Detailed discussion of all of these studies in detail is not permitted due to space constraints, but we highlight a few specific applications in which capture of particular structural characteristics of certain protein targets are facilitated by synthetic antibodies generated by in vitro display technology. In each case, such antibodies could not be obtained easily with traditional immunization approaches or from libraries based on natural immune repertories.

3.4.1 Engineering of Conformation-Specific Antibodies

One of the common approaches that nature utilizes for the regulation of protein function is protein allostery. For many signaling proteins, there exist multiple conformational states that mediate different cellular responses. Moreover, these conformational states are often dynamic and difficult to trap into one particular stable conformation. Antibodies that recognize a protein with one particular conformation state are powerful and highly sought-after for biological research, diagnostics, and therapeutics. In the in vivo system, a particular homogeneous protein conformation is difficult to maintain, which makes the generation of such antibodies by immunization complicated. In comparison, in vitro selection technologies can address these limitations by using negative selections to deplete nonspecific binders as well as those binders recognizing the nondesired protein conformation. If necessary, affinity maturation strategies can be applied for further specificity fine-tuning.

The key to successful development of conformation-specific antibodies is availability of the particular protein target in the appropriate conformation. Different strategies could be applied to bias distinct conformational states. One early study reported generation of scFvs specific to the GTP-bound form of the small GTPase Rab6 by performing selections with a GTP-locked mutant.[47] In another study, the protease caspase-1 was conformation-locked in either the active or inactive form by covalent linkage to small molecules. The locked antigens were then used to select Fabs that were highly selective for either of the two forms of the protease.[48] Antibodies from synthetic libraries have also been used to capture either the apo- or maltose-bound conformations of maltose-binding protein (MBP), providing reagents capable of discriminating between the two forms of the protein.[49] Structural characterization of a Fab bound to the closed form of MBP revealed an allosteric effect for increased ligand affinity (Fig. 3.4A). With the advent of cell suspension-based phage panning technology, development of antibodies discriminating between various conformational states of cell surface receptors in response to various stimuli or other physiological alterations has been investigated.[53]

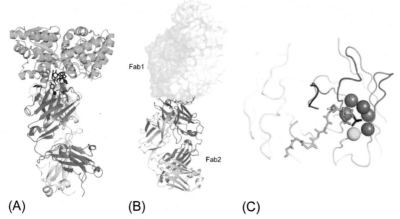

(A)   **(B)**   **(C)**

FIG. 3.4 Synthetic antibodies targeting conformational epitopes and PTMs. (A) Complex structure of a Fab (heavy chain, *deep gray*; light chain, *light gray*) that specifically recognizes the closed, maltose-bound form of MBP (*cyan*, PDB ID: 3PGF).[49] The maltose molecule is shown as sticks and colored *pink*. A set of aromatic residues within three VH CDRs, mostly in CDR-H3, are shown as sticks and colored *red*. These residues form the wedge structure that interacts with a region that is only exposed in the closed, maltose-bound conformation of MBP, hence conferring high conformational specificity. (B) Fab 309M3-B in complex with H3K9me3 peptide, the histone H3 peptide with trimethylated lysine residue (PDB ID: 4YHP).[50] Two identical 309M3-B Fabs, shown as Fab1 and Fab2, asymmetrically homodimerize with the peptide, which forms an expansive interface with one Fab bound to trimethylated Lys residue and the other to N-terminal histone. Fab 1 and Fab 2 are represented as surface or ribbon cartoons, respectively, with the light and heavy chains of the Fabs shown in *light gray* and *deep gray*, respectively. The H3K9me3 peptide is shown as sticks and colored *pink*, except for the trimethylated Lys residue which is colored *red*. (C) Design of biased antibody libraries targeting phosphorylated peptides. A natural antibody with an anion-binding nest in CDR-H2[51] was engineered to recognize phospho-serine (*pSer*), phospho-threonine (*pThr*), or phospho-tyrosine (*pTyr*) variants of an EGFRvIII peptide by phage selection. This design was derived from initial focused libraries with diversification introduced in CDR-H2 only.[52] The library configuration is represented by a Fab with crystal structure coordinates (PDB ID: 4JFZ). The framework is shown as *gray* tubes. The CDR-H2 residues selected for randomization are depicted as spheres. The phosphor-peptide is shown as sticks and colored *pink* with the exception of phosphoryl group in *red*. Using selected pSer- and pThr-specific antibodies identified from the initial libraries as templates, the second-generation libraries targeting pSer and pThr peptides were built with the conservation of the phosphor-residue-binding pocket in CDR-H2 and the introduction of diversification in selected residues of three CDR loops: CDR-L3 (*cyan*), CDR-H2 (*yellow*), and CDR-H3 (*blue*).

3.4.2 Engineering of Cross-Reactive Antibodies

Antigen recognition by mAbs is highly specific, and antibody engineering typically aims to achieve high specificity for a single antigen. However, under certain circumstances, defined cross-reactive antibodies are more powerful than monospecific counterparts. For example, cross-reactive antibodies that target orthologs of a particular target from different species (e.g., mouse, primate, and human) allow for better assessment of therapeutic efficacy and toxicity of the mAb in animal models. These antibodies are often difficult to obtain by hybridoma approaches due to immune tolerance. The in vitro nature of phage display technology with controlled selection processes makes development of cross-reactive antibodies readily achievable. For instance, human/mouse cross-reactive antibodies against highly conserved vascular endothelial growth factor (VEGF) have been obtained directly from naive synthetic antibody libraries.[4,54] For proteins that are less conserved between different species, cross-reactive antibodies can also be obtained by synthetic antibody engineering, as in the case of BAFF/BLyS receptor 3 (BR3) targeting antibody, in which highly cross-reactive antibody was evolved from initial antihuman antibodies with weak cross-reactivity to the mouse protein identified from naive libraries.[55]

In addition, cross-reactive antibodies against two closely related targets or even unrelated targets may provide synergistic therapeutic effects that cannot be obtained by simply mixing two monospecific antibodies against individual antigens. In this scenario, antibody engineering often involves enhancing dual specificity that involves preexisting weak recognition, due to homology between the targets. During the past few years, a series of "two-in-one" antibodies have been developed. This two-in-one antibody design provides an option for bispecific antibody therapeutics that can be manufactured in regular IgG or Fab formats. The first such antibody was developed in a proof-of-concept study; an antibody was evolved to recognize both its original antigen ErbB2 and VEGF, two proteins that are structurally unrelated but are frequently coexpressed in breast cancer (Fig. 3.5).[56] The "two-in-one" antibody was engineered to recognize both targets with affinities comparable to those of therapeutic antibodies, and it inhibited both VEGF- and ErbB2-mediated cell proliferation in vitro and tumor progression in mouse models.[57] Structural studies showed that the antibody binds the two antigens by using a common structural paratope, but the functional paratopes for ErbB2 and VEGF are located predominantly on VH or VL, respectively. As the expansion of this approach, an antibody that targeted epidermal growth factor receptor (EGFR) and ErbB3 was developed and shown to exhibit increased antitumor activity in a mouse model, compared with the respective monospecific Abs, and is now in clinical trials for treating epithelial-derived cancer.[58] More recently deep mutational scanning has been applied in antibody engineering to optimize the dual specificity binding site of a two-in-one antibody, and the resultant antibody achieved sub-nanomolar monovalent affinity against two structurally unrelated antigens such as VEGF and angiopoietin 2.[59]

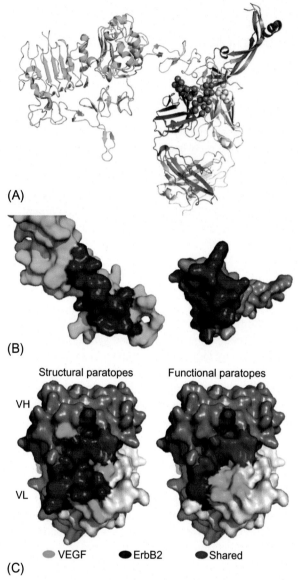

(A)

(B)

Structural paratopes   Functional paratopes

VH

VL

● VEGF   ● ErbB2   ● Shared

(C)

FIG. 3.5 A "two-in-one" antibody bH1 recognizes two distinct antigens ErbB2 and VEGF by differential engagement of VH and VL.[56] (A) Superposition of the bH1 Fab in complex with ErbB2 (PDB ID: 3BE1) or VEGF (PDB ID: 3BDY) bound to Fab bH1. All protein molecules are depicted in ribbons and colored as follows: bH1 VL, *light gray*; bH1 VH, *deep darker gray*; ErbB2, *cyan*; VEGF, *orange*. Spheres represent Fab residues belonging to CDR loops defined by the IMGT numbering Scheme.[38] (B) Surface representations of bH1-binding epitopes on ErbB2 (*left*) and VEGF (*right*) are shown in the same orientation relative to the Fab, demonstrating the distinct structural differences between the two epitopes. The residues in contact with bH1 (<4Å) are highlighted in *red*. (C) Comparison of structural and functional paratopes (CDR residues that contact antigen or energetically contribute to antigen binding, respectively) of bH1 for binding to ErbB2 or VEGF. On the surface of ErbB2-bound bH1 are color-mapped residues that make structural contacts (*left*) or energetic contributions (*right*) with ErbB2 (*blue*), VEGF (*green*), or both (*red*). The rest of the residues on the bH1 surface are colored either *deep gray* for VH or *light gray* for VL.

3.4.3 Engineering of Antibodies Specific for Point-Mutants and PTMs

Pathogenic viruses such as HIV and HBV frequently mutate to escape the host immune surveillance. In humans, single-nucleotide polymorphisms that result in an amino acid change in the encoded protein can be associated with genetic diseases or an altered susceptibility to disease. mAbs, with their exquisite epitope specificity, can be extremely useful in analysis of the mutant protein in virus or patient cells, which has been proven to be difficult largely due to the lack of mutation-specific detection tools. In addition to being powerful research tools to study infectious diseases, somatic and inherited genetic diseases, mAbs can also be applied as valuable medical tools for the diagnosis and prognosis of diseases as well as for therapeutic interventions. Hybridoma technology normally utilizes linear peptides harboring point residue mutation to immunize the animals, which is difficult to yield point-mutant targeting antibodies with high specificity and affinity. In contrast, in vitro selection approaches can direct selection pressure against the conformational epitope centered by the mutated residues so that both affinity and specificity can be optimized. If necessary, in vitro phage display-based antibody engineering can be applied to improve antibodies with desired properties. Through phage display and synthetic antibody engineering, antibodies that specifically target leucine to phenylalanine mutation at position 55 (L55F) on the major capsid viral protein 1 (VP1) of polyomavirus JC (JCV), a causative agent of progressive multifocal leukoencephalopathy (PML), were recently developed.[60] PML-specific mutations in JCV VP1 sequences, such as L55F and S269F, might favor PML onset. Initial selection from the naïve antibody library yielded an antibody with preferential recognition of L55F mutant vs the wild-type protein. One round of specificity fine-tuning based on homolog scanning analysis evolved antibodies with much higher specificity against L55F mutant. These L55F-specific antibodies could be potential candidates for developing tailored immune-based assays for PML risk stratification as well as research tools for the study of PML and JCV. This iterative process of point-mutant specific antibody development showcases the potential of synthetic antibody engineering, particularly with the emerging era of precision medicine and cancer immunotherapies.

In addition to developing point-mutant targeting antibodies, synthetic antibody technology has also been applied to identify antibodies recognizing proteins with PTMs. Similar to allostery, protein PTMs are responsible for many cellular activities. Specific reagents targeting particular PTMs are limited due to their ubiquitous and nonimmunogenic nature.

Of the various PTMs, histone PTMs are considered to be challenging targets for molecular recognition because of subtle differences among chemical moieties of PTMs, sequence similarity surrounding modification, and the fundamental challenge in recognizing flexible polypeptides due to unfavorable entropic changes associated with binding.[50,61] Currently available antihistone PTM antibodies went through limited validation and showed large lot-to-lot variation, which leads to low reproducibility in epigenetics research. Renewable recombinant antibodies highly specific to histone PTMs could fundamentally overcome this major limitation.[61] Recently recombinant antibodies were developed to target trimethylated lysine residues on histone H3.[50,61] First a single-chain Fv (scFv) clone was identified from a human naive antibody library that bound to trimethylated lysine with high specificity but low affinity and low sequence specificity. After extensive evolution based on shotgun-scanning mutagenesis analysis, one clone was identified, 309M3-A, that was highly specific for the histone 3 trimethyl lysine 9 modification (H3K9me3) binding with high affinity ($K_D = 24$ nM). The binding capacity 309M3-A was higher than that of the best available commercial antibody. More importantly, 309M3-A specifically recognized full-length histone H3 from human cell lines and performed well in standard epigenetics applications. After initial success in targeting H3K9me3, new antibodies to H3K9me3 and H3K4me3 were isolated, termed 309M3-B and 304M3-B, respectively. Crystal structures and biophysical analyses revealed an unprecedented mode of antibody-antigen recognition called "antigen clasping" (Fig. 3.4B), in which two antigen-binding sites of these antibodies form an unusual head-to-head dimer and cooperatively clasp the antigen in the dimer interface, thus rationalizing the high specificity.[50] These examples demonstrated that highly specific functional antibodies targeting PTMs could be obtained by the iterative process of recombinant antibody engineering and may lead to unique mechanisms of antigen recognition beyond the natural paradigm, a clear advantage of recombinant antibody development that is nearly impossible for conventional polyclonal and mAbs.

Phosphorylation is another major class of protein PTMs involved in cellular signaling. Therefore, tools that detect changes in phosphorylation state hold enormous value in biological research. Historically these phosphorylation-specific antibodies were obtained through animal immunization using phosphorylated peptide antigens. Unfortunately, naïve in vitro libraries rarely yield specific antibodies against phosphorylated peptide antigens due to similar reasons mentioned earlier regarding histone PTM-specific Abs, as well as the generalized design of naïve synthetic libraries. Recently, biased synthetic antibody libraries were described for isolating specific mAbs to phosphorylated peptide targets (Fig. 3.4C).[52] Guided by a natural phosphate-binding motif, a parent mAb scaffold was identified to engineer the designed pocket in CDRs. From combinatorial libraries constructed based on this scaffold, mAb scaffolds specific for phosphoserine, phosphothreonine, or phosphotyrosine were isolated. By selection with phage display antibody libraries constructed with structure-informed mutagenesis of these scaffolds, >50 phospho- and target-specific mAbs against 70% of phosphopeptide targets were generated. Hence this method holds great promise to be an effective design strategy for peptide targets with other PTMs.

3.5 CONCLUSIONS

mAbs serve as critical research, diagnostic, and therapeutic reagents, but a mAb performance and utility in these applications is a direct consequence of biochemical parameters (stability, affinity, and specificity). Although many approaches for the identification and optimization of mAbs exist, synthetic antibody engineering by phage display provides several advantages that have allowed isolation of unique reagents. Additional refinement of the current synthetic antibody libraries may be required in certain cases, but existing naïve libraries (e.g., Fig. 3.3) have shown remarkable applicability to a large number of antigens to date (>1000). As such, the agenda for the future will involve scaling the methodology and its particular application to new cases where traditional mAb approaches (e.g., hybridoma) have not been successful. Furthermore, the application of similar concepts and approaches to other protein scaffolds, such as non-antibody binding proteins or single domain monobodies, has been described extensively in the literature and has similar potential to provide novel reagents with high utility. Finally, the synthetic antibody design approach is predicated on both intrinsic biases inherent in natural immune repertoires, but also upon foundational knowledge of specific atomic factors that influence protein-protein interactions. Thus, efforts to further dissect and understand the basic physicochemical principles that govern antibody and protein-protein recognition are likely to continue to impact synthetic antibody design.

REFERENCES

1. Teillaud J.L., Desaymard C., Giusti A.M., Haseltine B., Pollock R.R., Yelton D.E., Zack D.J., Scharff M.D. Monoclonal antibodies reveal the structural basis of antibody diversity. *Science (New York, NY)* 1983;**222**:721–6.
2. Clackson T., Hoogenboom H.R., Griffiths A.D., Winter G. Making antibody fragments using phage display libraries. *Nature* 1991;**352**:624–8.
3. Fellouse F.A., Li B., Compaan D.M., Peden A.A., Hymowitz S.G., Sidhu S.S. Molecular recognition by a binary code. *J Mol Biol* 2005;**348**:1153–62.
4. Fellouse F.A., Wiesmann C., Sidhu S.S. Synthetic antibodies from a four-amino-acid code: a dominant role for tyrosine in antigen recognition. *Proc Natl Acad Sci U S A* 2004;**101**:12467–72.
5. Persson H., Ye W., Wernimont A., Adams J.J., Koide A., Koide S., Lam R., Sidhu S.S. CDR-H3 diversity is not required for antigen recognition by synthetic antibodies. *J Mol Biol* 2013;**425**:803–11.
6. Sidhu S.S., Fellouse F.A. Synthetic therapeutic antibodies. *Nat Chem Biol* 2006;**2**:682–8.
7. Colby D.W., Kellogg B.A., Graff C.P., Yeung Y.A., Swers J.S., Wittrup K.D. Engineering antibody affinity by yeast surface display. *Methods Enzymol* 2004;**388**:348–58.
8. Lipovsek D., Pluckthun A. In-vitro protein evolution by ribosome display and mRNA display. *J Immunol Methods* 2004;**290**:51–67.
9. Hornsby M., Paduch M., Miersch S., Saaf A., Matsuguchi T., Lee B., Wypisniak K., Doak A., King D., Usatyuk S., Perry K., Lu V., Thomas W., Luke J., Goodman J., Hoey R.J., Lai D., Griffin C., Li Z., Vizeacoumar F.J., Dong D., Campbell E., Anderson S., Zhong N., Graslund S., Koide S., Moffat J., Sidhu S., Kossiakoff A., Wells J. A high through-put platform for recombinant antibodies to folded proteins. *Mol Cell Proteomics* 2015;**14**:2833–47.

10. Nixon A.E., Sexton D.J., Ladner R.C. Drugs derived from phage display: from candidate identification to clinical practice. *MAbs* 2014;**6**:73–85.

11. Spiess C., Zhai Q., Carter P.J. Alternative molecular formats and therapeutic applications for bispecific antibodies. *Mol Immunol* 2015;**67**:95–106.

12. Gebleux R., Casi G. Antibody-drug conjugates: current status and future perspectives. *Pharmacol Ther* 2016;**167**:48–59.

13. Mazor Y., Van Blarcom T., Iverson B.L., Georgiou G. E-clonal antibodies: selection of full-length IgG antibodies using bacterial periplasmic display. *Nat Protoc* 2008;**3**:1766–77.

14. Sazinsky S.L., Ott R.G., Silver N.W., Tidor B., Ravetch J.V., Wittrup K.D. Aglycosylated immunoglobulin G1 variants productively engage activating Fc receptors. *Proc Natl Acad Sci U S A* 2008;**105**:20167–72.

15. MacCallum R.M., Martin A.C., Thornton J.M. Antibody-antigen interactions: contact analysis and binding site topography. *J Mol Biol* 1996;**262**:732–45.

16. Tomlinson I.M., Cox J.P., Gherardi E., Lesk A.M., Chothia C. The structural repertoire of the human V kappa domain. *EMBO J* 1995;**14**:4628–38.

17. Martin A., Scharff M.D. AID and mismatch repair in antibody diversification. *Nat Rev Immunol* 2002;**2**:605–14.

18. Patten P.A., Gray N.S., Yang P.L., Marks C.B., Wedemayer G.J., Boniface J.J., Stevens R.C., Schultz P.G. The immunological evolution of catalysis. *Science (New York, NY)* 1996;**271**:1086–91.

19. Wedemayer G.J., Patten P.A., Wang L.H., Schultz P.G., Stevens R.C. Structural insights into the evolution of an antibody combining site. *Science (New York, NY)* 1997;**276**:1665–9.

20. Yin J., Beuscher A.E.t., Andryski S.E., Stevens R.C., Schultz P.G. Structural plasticity and the evolution of antibody affinity and specificity. *J Mol Biol* 2003;**330**:651–656.

21. Li Y., Li H., Yang F., Smith-Gill S.J., Mariuzza R.A. X-ray snapshots of the maturation of an antibody response to a protein antigen. *Nat Struct Biol* 2003;**10**:482–8.

22. Birtalan S., Fisher R.D., Sidhu S.S. The functional capacity of the natural amino acids for molecular recognition. *Mol BioSyst* 2010;**6**:1186–94.

23. Smith G.P. Filamentous fusion phage—novel expression vectors that display cloned antigens on the virion surface. *Science* 1985;**228**:1315–7.

24. Kehoe J.W., Kay B.K. Filamentous phage display in the new millennium. *Chem Rev* 2005;**105**:4056–72.

25. Marks J.D., Hoogenboom H.R., Bonnert T.P., McCafferty J., Griffiths A.D., Winter G. Bypassing immunization—human-antibodies from v-gene libraries displayed on phage. *J Mol Biol* 1991;**222**:581–97.

26. Barbas C.F., Kang A.S., Lerner R.A., Benkovic S.J. Assembly of combinatorial antibody libraries on phage surfaces—the gene-III site. *Proc Natl Acad Sci U S A* 1991;**88**:7978–82.

27. Burton D.R., Barbas C.F., Persson M.A.A., Koenig S., Chanock R.M., Lerner R.A. A large array of human monoclonal-antibodies to type-1 human-immunodeficiency-virus from combinatorial libraries of asymptomatic seropositive individuals. *Proc Natl Acad Sci U S A* 1991;**88**:10134–7.

28. Vaughan T.J., Williams A.J., Pritchard K., Osbourn J.K., Pope A.R., Earnshaw J.C., McCafferty J., Hodits R.A., Wilton J., Johnson K.S. Human antibodies with sub-nanomolar affinities isolated from a large non-immunized phage display library. *Nat Biotechnol* 1996;**14**:309–14.

29. Giang E., Dorner M., Prentoe J.C., Dreux M., Evans M.J., Bukh J., Rice C.M., Ploss A., Burton D.R., Law M. Human broadly neutralizing antibodies to the envelope glycoprotein complex of hepatitis C virus. *Proc Natl Acad Sci U S A* 2012;**109**:6205–10.

30. Beerli R.R., Rader C. Mining human antibody repertoires. *MAbs* 2010;**2**:365–78.

31. Lee C.V., Liang W.C., Dennis M.S., Eigenbrot C., Sidhu S.S., Fuh G. High-affinity human antibodies from phage-displayed synthetic Fab libraries with a single framework scaffold. *J Mol Biol* 2004;**340**:1073–93.

32. Sidhu S.S., Li B., Chen Y., Fellouse F.A., Eigenbrot C., Fuh G. Phage-displayed antibody libraries of synthetic heavy chain complementarity determining regions. *J Mol Biol* 2004;**338**:299–310.

33. Knappik A., Ge L.M., Honegger A., Pack P., Fischer M., Wellnhofer G., Hoess A., Wolle J., Pluckthun A., Virnekas B. Fully synthetic human combinatorial antibody libraries (HuCAL) based on modular consensus frameworks and CDRs randomized with trinucleotides. *J Mol Biol* 2000;**296**:57–86.

34. Rauchenberger R., Borges E., Thomassen-Wolf E., Rom E., Adar R., Yaniv Y., Malka M., Chumakov I., Kotzer S., Resnitzky D., Knappik A., Reiffert S., Prassler J., Jury K., Waldherr D., Bauer S., Kretzschmar T., Yayon A., Rothe C. Human combinatorial Fab library yielding specific and functional antibodies against the human fibroblast growth factor receptor 3. *J Biol Chem* 2003;**278**:38194–205.

35. Rothe C., Urlinger S., Lohning C., Prassler J., Stark Y., Jager U., Hubner B., Bardroff M., Pradel I., Boss M., Bittlingmaier R., Bataa T., Frisch C., Brocks B., Honegger A., Urban M. The human combinatorial antibody library HuCAL GOLD combines diversification of all six CDRs according to the natural immune system with a novel display method for efficient selection of high-affinity antibodies. *J Mol Biol* 2008;**376**:1182–200.

36. Tiller T., Schuster I., Deppe D., Siegers K., Strohner R., Herrmann T., Berenguer M., Poujol D., Stehle J., Stark Y., Hessling M., Daubert D., Felderer K., Kaden S., Kolln J., Enzelberger M., Urlinger S. A fully synthetic human Fab antibody library based on fixed VH/VL framework pairings with favorable biophysical properties. *MAbs* 2013;**5**:445–70.

37. Fellouse F.A., Esaki K., Birtalan S., Raptis D., Cancasci V.J., Koide A., Jhurani P., Vasser M., Wiesmann C., Kossiakoff A.A., Koide S., Sidhu S.S. High-throughput generation of synthetic antibodies from highly functional minimalist phage-displayed libraries. *J Mol Biol* 2007;**373**:924–40.

38. Lefranc M.P., Pommie C., Ruiz M., Giudicelli V., Foulquier E., Truong L., Thouvenin-Contet V., Lefranc G. IMGT unique numbering for immunoglobulin and T cell receptor variable domains and Ig superfamily V-like domains. *Dev Comp Immunol* 2003;**27**:55–77.

39. Alt F.W., Blackwell T.K., Yancopoulos G.D. Development of the primary antibody repertoire. *Science* 1987;**238**:1079–87.

40. Tonegawa S. Somatic generation of antibody diversity. *Nature* 1983;**302**:575–81.

41. Koldobskaya Y., Duguid E.M., Shechner D.M., Suslov N.B., Ye J., Sidhu S.S., Bartel D.P., Koide S., Kossiakoff A.A., Piccirilli J.A. A portable RNA sequence whose recognition by a synthetic antibody facilitates structural determination. *Nat Struct Mol Biol* 2011;**18**:100–7.

42. Uysal S., Vásquez V., Tereshko V., Esaki K., Fellouse F.A., Sidhu S.S., Koide S., Perozo E., Kossiakoff A. Crystal structure of full-length KcsA in its closed conformation. *Proc Natl Acad Sci U S A* 2009;**106**:6644–9.

43. Uysal S., Cuello L.G., Cortes D.M., Koide S., Kossiakoff A.A., Perozo E. Mechanism of activation gating in the full-length KcsA K+ channel. *Proc Natl Acad Sci U S A* 2011;**108**:11896–9.

44. Koellhoffer J.F., Chen G., Sandesara R.G., Bale S., Saphire E.O., Chandran K., Sidhu S.S., Lai J.R. Two synthetic antibodies that recognize and neutralize distinct proteolytic forms of the Ebola virus envelope glycoprotein. *ChemBioChem* 2012;**13**:2549–57.

45. Kalb S.R., Garcia-Rodriguez C., Lou J.L., Baudys J., Smith T.J., Marks J.D., Smith L.A., Pirkle J.L., Barr J.R. Extraction of BoNT/A,/B,/E, and /F with a single, high affinity

monoclonal antibody for detection of botulinum neurotoxin by Endopep-MS. *PLoS One* 2010;**5**:e12237.

46. Garcia-Rodriguez C., Geren I.N., Lou J., Conrad F., Forsyth C., Wen W., Chakraborti S., Zao H., Manzanarez G., Smith T.J., Brown J., Tepp W.H., Liu N., Wijesuriya S., Tomic M.T., Johnson E.A., Smith L.A., Marks J.D. Neutralizing human monoclonal antibodies binding multiple serotypes of botulinum neurotoxin. *Protein Eng Des Sel* 2011;**24**:321–31.

47. Nizak C., Monier S., del Nery E., Moutel S., Goud B., Perez F. Recombinant antibodies to the small GTPase Rab6 as conformation sensors. *Science* 2003;**300**:984–7.

48. Gao J., Sidhu S.S., Wells J.A. Two-state selection of conformation-specific antibodies. *Proc Natl Acad Sci U S A* 2009;**106**:3071–6.

49. Rizk S.S., Paduch M., Heithaus J.H., Duguid E.M., Sandstrom A., Kossiakoff A.A. Allosteric control of ligand-binding affinity using engineered conformation-specific effector proteins. *Nat Struct Mol Biol* 2011;**18**:U437–69.

50. Hattori T., Lai D., Dementieva I.S., Montano S.P., Kurosawa K., Zheng Y.P., Akin L.R., Swist-Rosowska K.M., Grzybowski A.T., Koide A., Krajewski K., Strahl B.D., Kelleher N.L., Ruthenburg A.J., Koide S. Antigen clasping by two antigen-binding sites of an exceptionally specific antibody for histone methylation. *Proc Natl Acad Sci U S A* 2016;**113**:2092–7.

51. Landry R.C., Klimowicz A.C., Lavictoire S.J., Borisova S., Kottachchi D.T., Lorimer I.A.J., Evans S.V. Antibody recognition of a conformational epitope in a peptide antigen: Fv-peptide complex of an antibody fragment specific for the mutant EGF receptor, EGFRvIII. *J Mol Biol* 2001;**308**:883–93.

52. Koerber J.T., Thomsen N.D., Hannigan B.T., Degrado W.F., Wells J.A. Nature-inspired design of motif-specific antibody scaffolds. *Nat Biotechnol* 2013;**31**:916–21.

53. Eisenhardt S.U., Schwarz M., Bassler N., Peter K. Subtractive single-chain antibody (scFv) phage-display: tailoring phage-display for high specificity against function-specific conformations of cell membrane molecules. *Nat Protoc* 2007;**2**:3063–73.

54. Liang W.C., Wu X.M., Peale F.V., Lee C.V., Meng G., Gutierrez J., Fu L., Malik A.K., Gerber H.P., Ferrara N., Fuh G. Cross-species vascular endothelial growth factor (VEGF)-blocking antibodies completely inhibit the growth of human tumor xenografts and measure the contribution of stromal VEGF. *J Biol Chem* 2006;**281**:951–61.

55. Lee C.V., Hymowitz S.G., Wallweber H.J., Gordon N.C., Billeci K.L., Tsai S.P., Compaan D.M., Yin J.P., Gong O., Kelley R.F., DeForge L.E., Martin F., Starovasnik M.A., Fuh G. Synthetic anti-BR3 antibodies that mimic BAFF binding and target both human and murine B cells. *Blood* 2006;**108**:3103–11.

56. Bostrom J., Yu S.-F., Kan D., Appleton B.A., Lee C.V., Billeci K., Man W., Peale F., Ross S., Wiesmann C., Fuh G. Variants of the antibody herceptin that interact with HER2 and VEGF at the antigen binding site. *Science* 2009;**323**:1610–4.

57. Bostrom J., Haber L., Koenig P., Kelley R.F., Fuh G. High affinity antigen recognition of the dual specific variants of herceptin is entropy-driven in spite of structural plasticity. *PLoS One* 2011;**6**:e17887.

58. Schaefer G., Haber L., Crocker L.M., Shia S., Shao L., Dowbenko D., Totpal K., Wong A., Lee C.V., Stawicki S., Clark R., Fields C., Phillips G.D.L., Prell R.A., Danilenko D.M., Franke Y., Stephan J.P., Hwang J., Wu Y., Bostrom J., Sliwkowski M.X., Fuh G., Eigenbrot C. A two-in-one antibody against HER3 and EGFR has superior inhibitory activity compared with monospecific antibodies. *Cancer Cell* 2011;**20**:472–86.

59. Koenig P., Lee C.V., Sanowar S., Wu P., Stinson J., Harris S.F., Fuh G. Deep sequencing-guided design of a high affinity dual specificity antibody to target two Angiogenic factors in Neovascular age-related macular degeneration. *J Biol Chem* 2015;**290**:21773–86.

60. Chen G., Gorelik L., Simon K.J., Pavlenco A., Cheung A., Brickelmaier M., Chen L.L., Jin P., Weinreb P.H., Sidhu S.S. Synthetic antibodies and peptides recognizing progressive multifocal leukoencephalopathy-specific point mutations in polyomavirus JC capsid viral protein 1. *MAbs* 2015;**7**:681–92.

61. Hattori T., Taft J.M., Swist K.M., Luo H., Witt H., Slattery M., Koide A., Ruthenburg A.J., Krajewski K., Strahl B.D., White K.P., Farnham P.J., Zhao Y.M., Koide S. Recombinant antibodies to histone post-translational modifications. *Nat Methods* 2013;**10**:992–5.

Chapter 4

Natural Killer Cell Receptors

Sneha Rangarajan*,†, Roy A. Mariuzza*,†

*University of Maryland Institute for Bioscience and Biotechnology Research, Rockville, MD, United States, †University of Maryland, College Park, MD, United States

4.1 INTRODUCTION

Natural killer (NK) cells are innate lymphoid cells that participate in the elimination of tumor cells and virally infected cells.[1–3] The activation of NK cells is controlled by a dynamic interplay between positive signaling activating receptors and negative signaling inhibitory receptors.[4,5] The dominant signal, received by an NK cell through interaction with normal levels of major histocompatibility complex class I (MHC-I) molecules on target cells, is inhibitory. This inhibitory signal is attenuated—and the NK cell is activated—if tumorigenic or infectious processes reduce MHC-I expression.

NK receptors are members of two structural superfamilies: the immunoglobulin (Ig) superfamily and the C-type lectin superfamily.[6–8] Both superfamilies include inhibitory and activating receptors. In addition to MHC molecules, NK receptors recognize MHC-like and non-MHC molecules from both cellular and viral sources.

Inhibitory receptors specific for MHC-I include killer Ig-like receptors (KIRs) in humans, C-type lectin-like Ly49 receptors in rodents, leukocyte immunoglobulin-like receptors, and NKG2D/CD94 receptors.[2,5–8] Besides reduced inhibitory signals, activating signals are also necessary for NK cell triggering and target cell lysis.[3–5] These signals are transmitted by diverse activating receptors, including DNAM-1, NKG2D, and the natural cytotoxicity receptors (NCRs), whose ligands comprise both MHC-like and non-MHC molecules. The NCR family includes NKp30, NKp44, and NKp46. Additionally, a role for Ly49 receptors in viral immunity has been revealed by the interaction of activating Ly49s with gene products of mouse cytomegalovirus (MCMV).[9–11]

Besides NK receptors specific for classical or nonclassical MHC-I molecules, various other cell surface proteins have been implicated in the regulation of NK cytolytic activity.[2,5] These include NKR-P1,[12,13] NTB-A,[14,15] 2B4,[14–16] DNAM-1,[17] NKp30,[18] NKp44,[19] NKp46,[20] NKp65,[13,21] and NKp80,[13,22,23] which help control NK cell activation, and the inhibitory receptors LAIR-1[24]

Structural Biology in Immunology. https://doi.org/10.1016/B978-0-12-803369-2.00004-8

101

and KLRG1.[25,26] The natural ligands for most of these receptors have been identified, including CD48 for 2B4, CD155 for DNAM-1, B7-H6 for NKp30, KACL for NKp65, AICL for NKp80, collagen for LAIR-1, and E-cadherin for KLRG1.[2,5]

Remarkable progress has been made in determining crystal structures of representative NK receptors, both in free and ligand-bound forms. These structures collectively reveal that NK receptors have developed multiple strategies for recognizing diverse cellular and viral ligands, and thereby control NK cytotoxicity.

4.2 MHC-I RECOGNITION BY Ly49 RECEPTORS

The highly polymorphic Ly49 receptors, of which there are at least 23 members (Ly49A-W) in mice, are the main MHC-monitoring molecules on rodent NK cells.[27,28] Most Ly49s inhibit NK cell-mediated cytolysis upon binding MHC-I ligands.[27,29,30] However, some Ly49s are activating. Individual Ly49s recognize one or more H-2D and H-2K alleles.[27,29,30] Ly49s generally recognize MHC-I independently of the MHC-bound peptide. However, Ly49C and Ly49I display considerable peptide specificity.[31,32]

Ly49 receptors are members of the C-type lectin-like family of proteins although they do not have a functional calcium-binding site.[8] Ly49s are homodimeric type II transmembrane proteins. Each of their protein chains contains a C-type lectin-like domain (CTLD), known as the natural killer receptor domain (NKD). Each NKD within the Ly49 homodimer is linked to the transmembrane and cytoplasmic domains by a stalk of ~70 residues. Ly49s that are inhibitory transduce signals via immunoreceptor tyrosine-based inhibitory motifs (ITIM); by contrast, activating Ly49s utilize DAP12, the associated signaling molecule. DAP12 possesses an immunoreceptor tyrosine-based activation motif (ITAM).[5,27,29]

Researchers have determined crystal structures for: Ly49A NKD bound to H-2D[d33], Ly49C NKD bound to H-2K,[b34,35] Ly49C NKD,[33] Ly49I NKD,[34] Ly49G2 NKD,[33] Ly49L NKD,[35] Ly49L NKD with the stalk,[35] Ly49H in complex with the MCMV immunoevasin m157,[36] and Ly49C bound to the nonclassical MHC-Ib molecule H2-Q10.[37] Thanks to these studies, we now understand the molecular architecture of the MHC-binding site of Ly49 receptors, the way viral immunoevasins target Ly49s, and the mechanism of MHC-I engagement in *trans* and *cis*.

The Ly49 NKD possesses two α-helices (α1 and α2), as well as two antiparallel β-sheets that are formed by seven β-strands (Fig. 4.1A,C,E). Ly49s exist as dimers on the NK cell surface. These dimers may exist in two distinct conformations: "closed" and "open," as shown by Ly49A (Fig. 4.1A) and Ly49C (Fig. 4.1C,E), respectively. In the closed dimer conformation, the C-terminal ends of the α2 helices pack against one another, whereas in the open dimer the α2 helices are not juxtaposed. In the complex between Ly49A and H-2D[d] (Fig. 4.1A), the Ly49A homodimer uses just one of its subunits to complex with

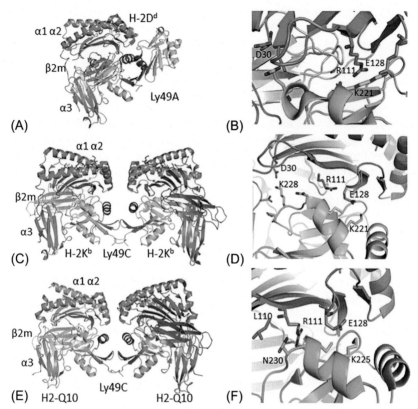

FIG. 4.1 Structures of Ly49-MHC-I complexes. (A) Ribbon diagram of Ly49A bound to H-2D^d (1QO3). The α1, α2, and α3 domains of the MHC-I heavy chain are *orange*; β$_2$m is *gray*; the peptide is magenta; the Ly49A dimer is *green*. The α2 helices of the Ly49A dimer are *red*. The complex is oriented with the H-2D^d molecule on the target cell at the bottom; the Ly49A homodimer reaches H-2D^d from an opposing NK cell at the top, to which it is connected via long stalk regions (not present in the crystal structure). (B) The Ly49A-H-2D^d interface. (C) Structure of Ly49C in complex with H-2K^b (3C8K). (D) The Ly49C-H-2K^b interface. (E) Structure of Ly49C in complex with H2-Q10 (5J6G). (F) The Ly49C-H2-Q10 interface. The side chains of contacting residues are drawn in ball-and-stick representation, with carbon atoms in *green* (Ly49A or Ly49C), *orange* (H-2D^d, H-2K^b, or H2-Q10), or *gray* (β$_2$m), oxygen atoms in *red*, and nitrogen atoms in *blue*.

one H-2D^d molecule; the site where this occurs is below the peptide-binding platform of the MHC-I ligand.[38] This site is formed by the α1/α2, α3, and β$_2$-microglobulin (β$_2$m) domains of H-2D^d and partially overlaps the binding site for CD8. By contrast, in the Ly49C-H-2K^b complex,[33,39] the Ly49C dimer engages H-2K^b bivalently, with each subunit contacting MHC-I at a site equivalent to the Ly49A binding site on H-2D^d (Fig. 4.1C). Ly49C interacts similarly with H2-Q10, which may play a role in regulating NK cell responses following cellular stress (Fig. 4.1E).[37]

The different geometries of the dimerization involving Ly49A and Ly49C explain the different types of MHC engagement in the Ly49A-H-2D^d and Ly49C-H-2K^b complexes. The Ly49A dimer in the closed conformation cannot bind two MHC ligands at the same time, as can occur with the open Ly49C dimer, because the result would be a spatial arrangement in which MHC molecules would clash. However, NMR analysis has shown that Ly49A predominantly adopts the open conformation in solution that can bind two MHC-I molecules.[40] Therefore, Ly49s most likely exist on the NK cell surface in dynamic equilibrium between closed and open forms. Ly49-mediated MHC-cross-linking by the closed form may enhance signal transduction by stabilizing receptor-ligand interactions at the NK cell-target cell interface.

Ly49s exhibit specificity for different MHC alleles. For example, whereas Ly49A and Ly49C only bind H-2D^d and H-2D^k, the promiscuous Ly49C recognizes H-2K^b, H-2K^d, H-2D^b, H-2D^d, and H-2D^k.[28,32] Specificity is conferred by residues 218–231, which exhibit high sequence variability across the Ly49 family.[33] This region adopts markedly different conformations in Ly49A (Fig. 4.1B) and Ly49C (Fig. 4.1D). Interactions at the Ly49C-H2-Q10 interface (Fig. 4.1F) mirror those in the Ly49C-H-2K^b interface (Fig. 4.1D), reflecting the conserved nature of these MHC molecules.[37]

Direct contacts between Ly49A and the peptide in the Ly49A-H-2D^d structure are completely absent, which explains why MHC recognition by Ly49A is independent of the sequence of the MHC-bound peptide (Fig. 4.1A).[38] By contrast, Ly49C displays remarkable peptide selectivity. This is difficult to understand in terms of the Ly49C-H-2K^b complex, which contains no contacts between Ly49C and peptide (Fig. 4.1C).[33,39] The biological role, if any, of the peptide selectivity of certain Ly49s (and KIRs; see below) is unknown.

4.3 Ly49 RECEPTORS INTERACT WITH MHC-I IN *TRANS* AND *CIS*

Cell surface receptors generally interact with ligands expressed on other cells in *trans* to mediate cell-to-cell communication. However, some cell surface receptors are known to bind ligands expressed on the same cell in *cis*.[41,42] These include Ly49 and LILR/PIR-B NK receptors, which interact with MHC-I molecules on opposing cells, as well as on the same cell.[43–45] Siglec-2 (CD22),[46,47] herpes virus entry mediator,[48] plexin receptors,[49] and Notch receptors[50,51] are also examples of cell surface receptors that act in both *trans* and *cis*. Such *cis* interactions serve to modulate (increase or decrease) the threshold at which a biological response[41,42] is produced due to cellular activation signaling.

Cis interactions that occur between Ly49 receptors and MHC-I promote NK cell activation by rendering them physically unavailable for functional *trans* interactions.[44,45] As a result, *cis* interactions improve the sensitivity of NK cells by lowering the threshold at which NK cell activation exceeds inhibition.[41] Moreover, *cis* interactions of Ly49A are necessary for NK cell education.[52]

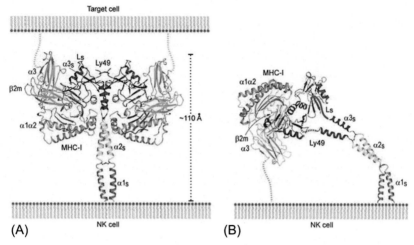

FIG. 4.2 Interaction of Ly49 receptors with MHC-I in *trans* and *cis*. (A) *Trans* interaction of an Ly49 homodimer on the NK cell with two MHC-I molecules on the target cell (3G8L). The α1, α2, and α3 domains of the MHC-I heavy chain are *cyan*; β2m is *green*; Ly49 NKD is *red*; helix α3$_S$ of the Ly49 stalk and loop L$_S$ connecting α3$_S$ to the NKD are *blue*; the disulfide bond linking the α3$_S$ helices is *magenta*. The α1$_S$ and α2$_S$ helices of the stalk are *orange* and *yellow*. To bind MHC-I in *trans*, the Ly49 stalks must assume a backfolded conformation. (B) *Cis* interaction of Ly49 with MHC-I. The Ly49 homodimer binds one MHC-I molecule on the NK cell itself. To bind MHC-I in *cis*, the Ly49 stalks must adopt an extended conformation. Reproduced with permission from *Immunity*.[35]

Trans and *cis* interactions utilize the same site to bind MHC-I.[44] As a result, to engage MHC-I in *trans* vs *cis*, Ly49 receptors must drastically reorient their NKDs relative to the NK cell membrane. The long stalk region of Ly49s provides the required flexibility. In the structure of Ly49L, the stalk is composed of α-helices and a loop of 12 residues connecting the helix to the NKD (Fig. 4.2A).[35] However, the Ly49L NKD is backfolded onto the NKD instead of projecting from the NKD. A model of the Ly49-MHC-I complex (Fig. 4.2A) shows that the N-termini of the stalks point in the opposite direction from the C-termini of the MHC-I molecules. Ly49s therefore assume the backfolded conformation so they can bind MHC-I in *trans*. For *cis* binding, these stalks assume an extended conformation that orients the NKDs with their N-termini toward the NK cell (Fig. 4.2B).

4.4 Ly49A'S RECOGNITION OF A VIRAL IMMUNOEVASIN

NK cells[53] directly recognize certain viral pathogens, as shown by studies of the susceptibility of different mouse strains to infection by MCMV. In C57BL/6 mice, resistance to infection is mediated by the activating receptor Ly49H, which impairs MCMV replication.[54-58] By contrast, BALB/c mice

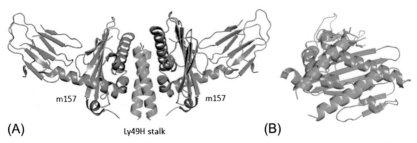

FIG. 4.3 Structure of the MCMV immunoevasin m157 bound to the Ly49H stalk. (A) Side view of the Ly49H-m157 complex (4JO8), in which two m157 monomers (*orange*) bind the helical Ly49H stalk (*green*). (B) Top view of the Ly49H-m157 complex, in which the Ly49H stalk lies across the α1/α2 platform of m157.

lack a gene for Ly49H and do not restrict MCMV replication. Ly49H binds directly to the MHC-I homolog m157,[59] a viral glycoprotein expressed on MCMV-infected cells.[9,10]

X-ray crystallography studies have shown that m157 binds to the stalk region of Ly49H and not to the NKDs, which recognize MHC-I.[36] m157 was well resolved in the Ly49H-m157 structure, but only the α-helices of Ly49H could be seen within the electron density (Fig. 4.3A). Mutagenesis studies revealed that binding to m157 occurred entirely through the Ly49H stalk and that the interaction[36] involved no contribution from the NKD. In the Ly49H-m157 complex, two m157 monomers engage the Ly49H dimer in such a way that the stalks straddle the α1/α2 platform of m157 (Fig. 4.3B). The ability of m157 to target-specific members of the Ly49 family correlates with sequence differences in the stalk region.[36] The recognition mode in the Ly49H-m157 complex is not possible unless Ly49 is in the extended state, which is the same conformation that recognizes MHC-I in *cis* (Fig. 4.2B). The Ly49H stalk segment would not be accessible to m157 in the backfolded conformation (Fig. 4.2A). Biophysical measurements showed that conformational selection is involved in binding, and that only the extended conformation of Ly49H can bind a first m157 ligand, which is then followed by the binding of a second m157 ligand.[60]

4.5 RECOGNITION OF MHC-I BY KIR RECEPTORS

The KIR receptor family is highly polymorphic and constitutes the main MHC-monitoring molecules found on primate NK cells. Inhibitory and activating receptors both belong to the KIR family. KIRs are type I transmembrane glycoproteins that have two (D1 and D2; designated KIR2D) or three (D0, D1, and D2; designated KIR3D) extracellular C2-type Ig-like domains.[6,8] Whereas KIR3D receptors recognize HLA-A and HLA-B alleles, KIR2D receptors recognize HLA-C alleles. The specificity of KIR2D receptors for HLA-C has been addressed through crystallographic studies of KIR2D molecules, both in unbound form[61–65] and in complex with HLA-C ligands.[66,67] The basis for

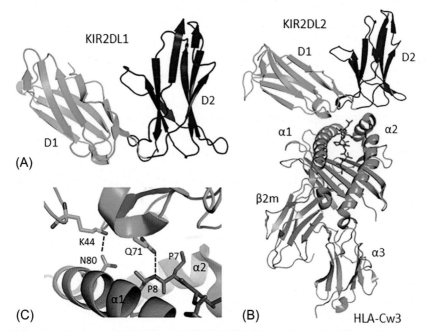

FIG. 4.4 Structures of KIR2DL and KIR2DL-HLA-C complexes. (A) Ribbon diagram of KIR2DL1 (1NKR). The D1 domain is *green*; D2 is *blue*. (B) Ribbon diagram of KIR2DL2 bound to HLA-Cw3 (1EFX). The α1, α2, and α3 domains of the HLA-Cw3 heavy chain are *orange*; β2m is *gray*; the peptide is *magenta*. (C) Basis for allelic specificity and peptide selectivity of KIR2D receptors. The dotted lines represent hydrogen bonds formed by HLA-Cw3 Asn80 with KIR2DL2 Lys44, and by HLA-Cw3 Gln71 with residue P8 of the peptide.

MHC-I recognition by three-domain KIRs[68] has been revealed by the structure of KIR3DL1 bound to HLA-B*5701.

KIR2D receptors comprise two tandem Ig-like domains (D1 and D2) connected by a linker of 3–5 amino acids (Fig. 4.4A). In the KIR2DL2-HLA-Cw3[66] and KIR2DL1-HLA-Cw4[67] complexes, the KIRs bind HLA-C through the α1 and α2 helices and the C-terminus of the peptide (Fig. 4.4B). The D1D2 axis is orthogonal to the axis of the bound peptide and the HLA-C α1 helix. This binding mode is completely distinct from that of Ly49 NK receptors (Fig. 4.1A,C). Each KIR contacts the α1 and α2 helices of HLA-C through six loops in its interdomain hinge region.

The KIR2DL2-HLA-Cw3[66] and KIR2DL1-HLA-Cw4[67] structures explain the allelic specificity of KIR2DLs. With one exception (Asn80), all HLA-Cw3 residues in contact with KIR2DL2 are invariant in all HLA-C alleles, including HLA-Cw4. Mutagenesis has shown that Asn80 is essential for defining allelic specificity. Among the KIR2DL2 residues that contact HLA-Cw3, the only ones that differ in KIR2DL1 are those at positions 44 and 70. In the KIR2DL2-HLA-Cw3 structure, KIR2DL2 Lys44 forms a hydrogen bond with HLA-Cw3

Asn80 (Fig. 4.4C). This hydrogen bond would not be able to form if Lys44 were replaced by methionine, as in KIR2DL1. The side chain of HLA-Cw4 Lys80 in the KIR2DL1-HLA-Cw4 complex is located in a negatively charged pocket that includes KIR2DL1 Met44. If, as in KIR2DL2, Met44 were to be replaced by lysine, the result would be charge repulsion with HLA-Cw4 Lys80, which would cause binding to be lost.

As in the case of Ly49s (see earlier), peptide preferences have been documented in KIR2D binding to HLA-C molecules,[69,70] although it remains to be established whether peptide selectivity is involved in NK receptor function. In this regard, KIR-associated HIV-1 sequence polymorphisms in chronically infected individuals reduce the antiviral activity of KIR-positive NK cells, possibly by enhancing the binding of inhibitory KIRs to HIV-1-infected CD4$^+$ T cells.[71] The KIR-HLA interaction is most sensitive to substitutions at peptide positions P7 and P8, in agreement with the KIR2DL2-HLA-Cw3 and KIR2DL1-HLA-Cw4 structures.[66,67]

In the KIR3DL1-HLA-B*5701 complex,[68] KIR3DL1 binds to HLA-B*5701 with its D1 and D2 domains positioned over the C-terminal end of the peptide-binding groove—an orientation that resembles the KIR2D-HLA-C complexes (Fig. 4.5A). KIR3DL1 assumes an extended conformation that enables D0 to project toward β_2m and bind a site on HLA-B*5701 that is highly conserved across HLA-A and HLA-B allotypes. The D1 domain makes contact with the α1 helix and the self-peptide; the D2 domain makes contact with the α2 helix. More specifically, the D2 domain engages primarily with HLA-B*5701 residues 142–151. Those residues display limited polymorphism among HLA-B alleles (Fig. 4.5B). KIR3DL1 recognizes HLA allotypes that contain the Bw4 epitope-defining residues 77–83 on the α1 helix. In the structure,[68] KIR3DL1 makes contact through its D1 domain with residues 79, 80, and 83 within the Bw4 epitope (Fig. 4.5C), thereby explaining the allelic specificity of KIR3DLs. Surprisingly, the extensive polymorphisms that occur within individual KIR3D families are primarily situated at positions not directly involved in HLA binding. Nevertheless, these polymorphisms have the potential for indirectly affecting HLA binding by changing the expression levels or the clustering of KIR3D receptors found on the NK cell surface.

4.6 RECOGNITION OF MHC-I BY LILRs

The human LILR family of immunoreceptors is found on NK cells, T cells, monocytes, B cells, and dendritic cells.[72] Paired immunoglobulin receptors (PIRs) are the mouse orthologs of LILRs. LILRs resemble KIRs in that they possess either two or four tandem extracellular Ig-like domains. LILRA1, LILRA2, LILRA3, LILRB1, and LILRB2 bind HLA-A, -B, and -C. By contrast, several other LILRs—LILRA4, LILRA5, LILRA6, LILRB3, and LILRB4— apparently do not recognize MHC-I molecules. Besides acting as MHC-I sensors, LILRs may participate in the immune system's response to infection by

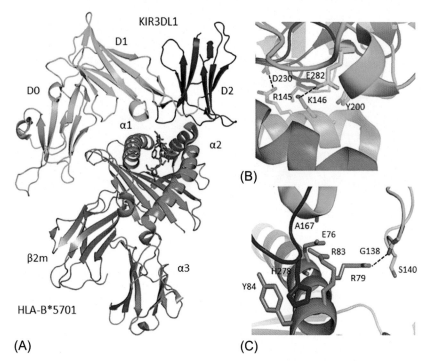

FIG. 4.5 Structure of the KIR3DL1-HLA-B*5701 complex. (A) Ribbon diagram of KIR3DL1 bound to HLA-B*5701 (3VH8). The HLA-B*5701 heavy chain is *orange*; β2m is *gray*; the peptide is *magenta*. The KIR3DL1 D0 domain is *cyan*; D1 is *green*; D2 is *blue*. (B) Contacts between KIR3DL1 and the HLA-B*5701 α2 helix. The D2 domain mainly interacts with HLA-B*5701 residues 142–151, which display limited polymorphism among HLA-B alleles. (C) Contacts between KIR3DL1 and the HLA-B*5701 α1 helix. KIR3DL1 recognizes HLA allotypes that contain the Bw4 epitope-defining residues 77–83 on the α1 helix.

viruses.[73] Structures of LILRB1 have been reported in unliganded form,[74] and bound to HLA-A2[75] and UL18, a MHC-I mimic encoded by human cytomegalovirus (HCMV).[76] Structures have also been determined for LILRB2 in free form[77] and in complex with HLA-G.[78]

The two tandem Ig-like domains (D1 and D2) of both LILRB1 and LILRB2 form a bent structure (Fig. 4.6A), similar to KIR2D (Fig. 4.4A). In the LILRB1-HLA-A2 complex,[75] LILRB1 D1D2 binds the HLA-A2 α3 domain, which is relatively nonpolymorphic, and β2m, which is invariant. LILRB1 D1 contacts the HLA-A3 α3 domain, while the D1–D2 interdomain hinge region contacts β2m (Fig. 4.6A). LILRB2 recognizes the HLA-G α3 in a similar fashion.[78] This docking mode differs completely from that of KIRs (Fig. 4.4B). The focus by LILRs on conserved elements of MHC-I molecules explains their broad specificity for numerous HLA alleles.

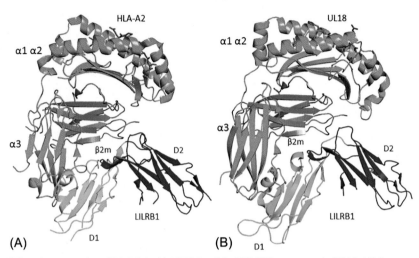

FIG. 4.6 Interaction of LILRB1 with MHC-I and the HCMV immunoevasin UL18. (A) Structure of LILRB1 bound to HLA-A2 (1P7Q). The α1, α2, and α3 domains of the HLA-A2 heavy chain are *orange*; β2m is *gray*; the peptide is *magenta*. The D1 and D2 domains of LILRB1 are *green* and *blue*, respectively. (B) Structure of LILRB1 in complex with the HCMV MHC-I mimic UL18 (3D2U).

4.7 LILR RECOGNITION OF THE VIRAL IMMUNOEVASIN UL18

Proteins synthesized by cytomegaloviruses hamper recognition by both NK cells and T cells and interfere with antigen processing and presentation.[79–81] Among these immunoevasins are several proteins that are structural homologs of host MHC-I molecules. UL18, the MHC-I mimic encoded by HCMV, binds the inhibitory receptor LILRB1.[82] As a result, HCMV-infected cells are able to escape NK cell-mediated lysis.[83] The decoy ligand UL18 associates with β2m[84] and is a heavily glycosylated transmembrane protein that binds LILRB1 > 1000-fold more tightly than MHC-I proteins. As a result, UL18 is in competition with MHC-I for binding to LILRB1.[85]

Although UL18 only shares ~25% sequence identity with MHC-I molecules, the structure of the UL18-LILRB1 complex is remarkably similar to those of the LILRB1-HLA-A2 and LILRB2-HLA-G complexes. The LILRB1 D1 domain contacts the UL18 α3 domain and the D1–D2 interdomain hinge contacts β2m (Fig. 4.6B).[76] Variable residues in the UL18 α1 domain do not contact LILRB1. Better surface complementarity and extra salt bridges found at the LILRB1-UL18 interface compared with the LILRB1-HLA-A2 interface are the probable reason for the >1000-fold higher affinity of UL18.

4.8 NATURAL CYTOTOXICITY RECEPTORS

In humans, the NCR family includes NKp46 (CD335), NKp44 (CD336), and NKp30 (CD337).[86] These powerful activating receptors are type I transmembrane glycoproteins comprising one (NKp46, NKp30) or two (NKp44) Ig-like extracellular domains.[86,87] NCRs possess charged residues in their transmembrane regions for interaction with ITAM-bearing signaling polypeptides: DAP12 for NKp44 and ζ-γ for NKp46 and NKp30.[88] NCRs are important in enabling NK cells to lyse diverse tumor cells, including neuroblastomas, carcinomas, and lymphoblastic and myeloid leukemias.[86,87] NCRs have also been implicated in protective responses against various viruses.[89–92]

Ligands for the NRC family have proven very elusive, but some progress has been made in identifying them. The receptors NKp44 and NKp46 bind influenza and other viral hemagglutinins (HAs). They do so by recognizing the HA of sialic acid moieties on N-linked glycans of these NCRs.[89,93] Binding of NKp46 to heparan sulfate proteoglycans has also been reported.[94] One cellular ligand for NKp44[95] is a novel isoform of the mixed-lineage leukemia-5 protein (MLL5). This MLL5 isoform was detected on tumor cell lines but is not expressed on normal cells.

NKp30 recognizes the tegument pp65 protein of HCMV,[96] the nuclear factor BAT3,[97] and the stress-induced cell surface protein B7-H6.[98] B7-H6 is a member of the B7 family. This family of immunoregulatory ligands includes ligands (B7-1 and B7-2) for the T cell costimulatory receptor CD28 and the coinhibitory receptor CTLA-4, as well as ligands (PD-L1 and PD-L2) for the T cell coinhibitory receptor PD-1.[99] Normal human tissues do not express B7-H6, but it is selectively expressed on stressed cells, including a wide variety of tumors, such as melanomas, T and B lymphomas, neuroblastomas, and carcinomas.[98,100–102] The interaction of B7-H6 on tumor cells with NKp30 on NK cells results in interferon-γ production and tumor cell killing. Thus, B7-H6 functions as a tumor-induced self-molecule that alerts innate immunity to cellular transformation.[98,100–102]

Structures have been described for NKp30, NKp44, and NKp46 in unbound form[103–105] and for NKp30 bound to B7-H6.[106] NKp44 consists of a single V-type Ig-like domain. Its main feature is an electropositive groove, which is formed by two facing β-hairpin loops that project from the Ig fold core (Fig. 4.7A).[103] This groove may be a possible binding site for anionic ligands, such as sialic acid. The receptor NKp46 consists of two C2-set Ig-like domains whose spatial arrangement resembles the KIR and LILR D1D2 domains (Fig. 4.7B).[104]

The Ig-like domain of NKp30 exhibits the chain topology found in C1-set domains (Fig. 4.7C).[105,106] The closest structural homolog of NKp30 is the V-like domain of PD-L1, a ligand for the T cell inhibitory receptor PD-1.[99] Like other members of the B7 family, B7-H6 is composed of a membrane-distal V-like domain and a membrane-proximal C-like domain.[106] The structure of the NKp30-B7-H6 complex revealed an assembly with a 1:1 receptor-ligand stoichiometry and a binding interface formed by the front and back β-sheets of the NKp30 C-like domain and the front β-sheet of the B7-H6 V-like domain (Fig. 4.7C).[106] B7-H6 contacts NKp30 in an antibody-like manner. In particular, the FG loop of the B7-H6 V-like domain corresponds to the complementarity-determining region (CDR) 3 of antibodies. It forms a prominent bulge on the surface of the ligand that fits snugly into a groove on NKp30. Residues from

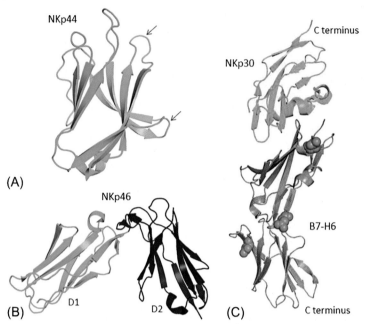

FIG. 4.7 Natural cytotoxicity receptors. (A) Structure of NKp44 (1HKF). The CC' and FG loops, marked with red arrows, define a positively charged groove that may bind anionic ligands. (B) Structure of NKp46 (1P6F). D1 is *green*; D2 is *blue*. (C) Structure of NKp30 bound to the stress-induced cellular ligand B7-H6 (3PV6). N-linked glycans at B7-H6 residues Asn43 and Asn57 in the V-like domain and Asn208 in the C-like domain are shown as *cyan spheres*.

the BC (CDR1-like) and C'C″ (CDR2-like) loops of B7-H6 provide additional contacts. It remains to be determined how NKp30 binds HCMV pp65[96] and BAT3.[97]

4.9 LIGAND BINDING BY NKG2D

NKG2D is expressed on NK cells and cytotoxic T cells and is a homodimeric C-type lectin-like receptor. This receptor recognizes several of MHC-I's structural homologs, including MICA, MICB, ULBP1–3, and RAE-1β, all of which lack a peptide-binding groove and β$_2$m.[107,108] In humans, MICA and MICB are upregulated in tumors and stressed cells compared to normal tissues.[109,110] RAE-1, MULT-1, and H-60 are upregulated in tumor cells of rodents but not in normal rodent cells.[111,112] These differential expression patterns indicate that NKG2D functions as a key receptor for NK cells as they conduct tumor surveillance. In mice, the MCMV-encoded immunoevasins m145, m152, and m155 downregulate expression of MULT-1, RAE-1, and H60, respectively, thereby evading NKG2D-mediated antiviral responses.[81,113] By binding the NKG2D ligands MICB, ULBP1, and ULBP2,[114] the HCMV-encoded immunoevasin UL16 acts as a decoy

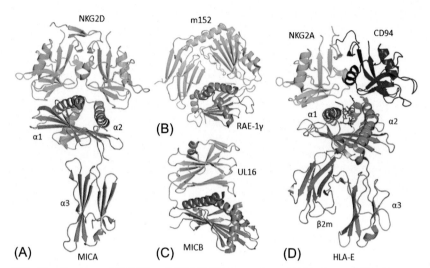

FIG. 4.8 Structures of NKG2D and NKG2A/CD94 complexes. (A) The human NKG2D-MICA complex (1HYR). The NKG2D homodimer is *green*; MICA is *orange*. (B) Structure of the MCMV immunoevasin m152 bound to the NKG2D ligand RAE-1γ (4G59). (C) Structure of the HCMV immunoevasin UL16 bound to MICB (2WY3). (D) The human NKG2A/CD94-HLA-E complex (3CDG). The NKG2A and CD94 subunits of the NKG2A/CD94 heterodimer are *green* and *blue*, respectively.

receptor. Research has solved the structures for human and mouse NKG2D in un-bound form,[115,116] for human NKG2D bound to MICA and ULBP3,[108,117] and for mouse NKG2D bound RAE-1β.[118] Structures have also been reported for m152 in complex with RAE-1γ,[113] and for UL16 bound to MICB.[114]

MICA is composed of an α1/α2 platform domain. This domain contains the α1 and α2 helices, which define the peptide-binding groove in classical MHC-I molecules, and also an Ig-like α3 domain (Fig. 4.8A).[119] The NKG2D homodimer engages MICA orthogonally to the α1 and α2 helices of the platform domain.[117] The symmetric NKG2D receptor's recognition of the asymmetric MICA ligand is facilitated by similar sites on the NKG2D monomers, which contact distinct sites on MICA. NKG2D binds ULBP3 and RAE-1β orthogonally to the α1/α2 domain of these MHC-like ligands, in a manner similar to the NKG2D-MICA complex.[108,118] These studies have revealed NKG2D's remarkable ability to use a single binding site to recognize MICA, ULBP3, and RAE-1β, even though these ligands have only about 25% of their amino acid sequences in common.

In the MCMV m152-RAE-1γ complex,[113] the MHC-I-like immunoevasin binds the α1 and α2 helices of RAE-1γ in a pincerlike manner that is similar to the interaction between NKG2D and MICA (Fig. 4.8B). By contrast, the Ig-like UL16 protein binds quite differently. It uses a three-stranded β-sheet to engage the α1 and α2 helices of MICB (Fig. 4.8C). Through their competition with NKG2D, m152 and UL16 prevent NKG2D-mediated NK cell activation that would kill viruses.[120–122]

4.10 HLA-E RECOGNITION BY NKG2/CD94

In addition to the homodimeric NKG2D receptor, the NKG2D family includes the receptors NKG2A, NKG2B, NKG2C, and NKG2E, which form heterodimers with CD94.[123–125] NKG2A and NKG2B act as inhibitory receptors; NKG2C and NKG2E function as activating receptors. The nonclassical MHC-I molecule HLA-E is the ligand for NKG2/CD94 receptors. It binds peptides derived from the leader peptides of classical and nonclassical MHC-I proteins.[123–125] HLA-E does not express on the cell surface without a bound peptide, so its expression depends on the production of other MHC-I molecules. In this way, HLA-E recognition by NKG2/CD94 enables NK cells to monitor expression of other MHC-I molecules on target cells.

NKG2A/CD94's structure has been determined in free form[126] and bound to HLA-E bearing a peptide from the HLA-G leader sequence.[127,128] NKG2A/CD94 straddles HLA-E's peptide-binding groove, with the NKG2A and CD94 subunits in contact with the α2 and α1 helices of HLA-E, respectively (Fig. 4.8D). The invariant CD94 subunit, rather than NKG2A,[127,128] contributes most of the buried surface area in the NKG2A/CD94-HLA-E complex. CD94 also dominates interactions with the peptide and is positioned over the P8 residue. NKG2A/CD94's focus on the C-terminal half of the peptide is worth noting because almost all of the sequence variation among HLA-*E*-restricted peptides is concentrated there.

4.11 RECOGNITION OF CADHERINS BY KLRG1

Killer cell lectin-like receptor G1 (KLRG1) is a C-type lectin-like inhibitory receptor. It is present on between 50% and 80% of human NK cells. Following infection with viruses or parasites,[129–134] KLRG1's expression is highly upregulated. E-cadherin[25,26,135] is the biological ligand for KLRG. E-cadherin establishes tight binding between neighboring epithelial cells in adherens junctions.[136] E-cadherin comprises five Ig-like extracellular domains (EC1–EC5). KLRG1 also recognizes N- and R-cadherins.[25] The binding of E-cadherin to KLRG1 wards off tissue damage[25,88,137] by preventing E-cadherin-expressing epithelial cells from being lysed by KLRG1$^+$ NK cells. In addition, KLRG1 may play a role in tumor immunosurveillance by detecting epithelial tumors with downregulated E-cadherin expression, which renders them metastatic.[137–139]

In the structure of KLRG1 bound to the EC1 domain of E-cadherin, one KLRG1 CTLD engages one EC1 molecule (Fig. 4.9).[140] KLRG1's recognition of its non-MHC ligand resembles Ly49 recognition of MHC-I, where each CTLD subunit contains an entire ligand-binding site (Fig. 4.1C). By contrast, NKG2D and MICA[117] bind at a site formed by two CTLD monomers (Fig. 4.8A). E-cadherin binds to a surface of KLRG1 that resembles the ligand-binding site of Ly49s and other C-type lectin-like NK receptors.[140] KLRG1 interacts primarily with residues Val3-Ile7 of E-cadherin, which are stringently conserved in E-, N-, and R-cadherins. As a result, NK cells bearing a single KLRG1 receptor can monitor target cells for the expression of different cadherins.

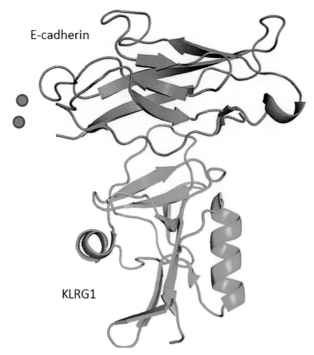

FIG. 4.9 Cadherin recognition by KLRG1. Structure of KLRG1 bound to the membrane-distal D1 domain of E-cadherin (3FF8). KLRG1 is *green* and E-cadherin is *orange*. Bound Ca²⁺ ions are drawn as *blue spheres*.

4.12 C-TYPE LECTIN-LIKE RECEPTOR-LIGAND PAIRS IN THE NK GENE COMPLEX

The NK gene complex (NKC) encodes approximately 30 cell surface glyco-proteins of the C-type lectin-like superfamily.[141] NKC genes can be subdivided into two types: killer cell lectin-like receptor (KLR) genes and C-type lectin receptor (CLEC) genes. KLR genes encode molecules that are expressed on NK cells, whereas CLEC genes encode molecules that are expressed on other types of cells. Members of the KLR family include NKG2D, NKG2A/CD94, and Ly49s, which bind MHC-I or MHC-related molecules (see earlier). Other members of the KLR family are receptors that do not engage ligands with an MHC-like fold (e.g., KLRG1-E-cadherin) (Fig. 4.9), as well as receptors that interact with CLEC2 glycoproteins that are themselves members of the C-type lectin-like superfamily.[13] These KLR and CLEC2 molecules, whose genes are intermingled in the NKC, function as genetically linked receptor-ligand pairs to modulate (promote or prevent) NK cell-mediated cytotoxicity. These pairs include Nkrp1-Clr,[142,143] NKRP1A-LLT1,[144–147]

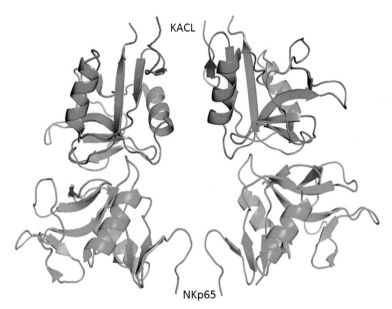

FIG. 4.10 KACL recognition by NKp65. Structure of the NKC-encoded human NKp65-KACL complex (4IOP). NKp65 is *green* and the KACL dimer is *orange*.

NKp80-AICL,[13,23,148] and NKp65-KACL.[13,21,149] Structures have been determined for unbound forms of mouse Clr,[150] mouse Nkrp1,[151] and human LLT1,[152] revealing homodimers whose subunits adopt the CTLD fold. However, only one complex structure, that of NKp65 bound to KACL, has been reported so far (Fig. 4.10).[153]

NKp65 stimulates NK cytotoxicity and release of proinflammatory cytokines upon binding KACL on keratinocytes, indicating that the NKp65-KACL pair serves a dedicated role in the immune surveillance of human skin.[13,21,149] Whereas KACL forms a homodimer resembling the NKG2D and Ly49 homodimers, NKp65 is monomeric.[153] In the NKp65-KACL complex, the KACL homodimer engages NKp65 bivalently, with each KACL subunit constituting an independent binding site for NKp65 and each NKp65 molecule making identical contacts with KACL (Fig. 4.10).

A mutational analysis of KACL residues in contact with NKp65 identified several "hot spot" residues that are critical for binding.[153] Importantly, these hot spot residues are strictly conserved or conservatively substituted among KACL, AICL, Clr, and LLT1. Furthermore, they come in contact with residues on NKp65, NKp80, Nkrp1, and NKRP1A, which themselves are strictly or highly conserved. As a result, the docking mode seen in the NKp65-KACL complex is probably similar to other NKC-encoded receptor-ligand pairs, including NKp80-AICL, Nkrp1-Clr, and NKRP1A-LLT1.

4.13 PERSPECTIVE

The structural studies described in this chapter have provided atomic-level insights into how representative NK receptors recognize cellular and viral ligands. This information provides a solid framework for understanding how NK cells discriminate between normal and tumor or virus-infected cells of the host. Two important mechanisms remain to be discovered: the biophysical mechanism by which inhibitory or activating signals are transmitted to the NK cell following ligand binding, and precisely how NK cells integrate these opposing signals to ultimately determine the outcome of encounters with target cells. Further research on membrane-embedded NK receptors and their associated signaling molecules should yield vital information needed to link ligand recognition and NK cell function.

REFERENCES

1. Di Santo JP. Natural killer cells: diversity in search of a niche. *Nat Immunol* 2008;**9**(475):473.
2. Vivier E, Tomasello E, Baratin M, Walzer T, Ugolini S. Functions of natural killer cells. *Nat Immunol* 2008;**9**:503–10.
3. Vivier E, Raulet DH, Moretta A, Caligiuri MA, Zitvogel L, Lanier LL, et al. Innate or adaptive immunity? The example of natural killer cells. *Science* 2011;**331**:44–9.
4. Lanier LL. Up on the tightrope: natural killer cell inhibition and activation. *Nat Immunol* 2008;**9**:495–502.
5. Long EO, Sik KH, Liu D, Peterson ME, Rajagopalan S. Controlling natural killer cell responses: integration of signals for activation and inhibition. *Annu Rev Immunol* 2013;**31**: 227–58.
6. Joyce MG, Sun PD. The structural basis of ligand recognition by natural killer cell receptors. *J Biomed Biotech* 2011;**2011**:203628.
7. Finton KA, Strong RK. Structural insights into activation of antiviral NK cell responses. *Immunol Rev* 2012;**250**:239–57.
8. Li Y, Mariuzza RA. Structural basis for recognition of cellular and viral ligands by NK cell receptors. *Front Immunol* 2014;**5**:123.
9. Arase H, Mocarski ES, Campbell AE, Hill AB, Lanier LL. Direct recognition of cytomegalovirus by activating and inhibitory NK cell receptors. *Science* 2002;**296**:1323–6.
10. Smith HR, Heusel JW, Mehta IK, Kim S, Dorner BG, Naidenko OV, et al. Recognition of a virus-encoded ligand by a natural killer cell activation receptor. *Proc Natl Acad Sci U S A* 2002;**99**:8826–31.
11. Derosiers M-P, Kielczewska A, Loredi-Osti J-C, Adam SG, Makrigiannis AP, Lemiex S, et al. Epistasis between mouse Klra and major histocompatibility complex class I loci is associated with a new mechanism of natural killer cell-mediated innate resistance to cytomegalovirus infection. *Nat Genet* 2005;**37**:593–9.
12. Plougastel BF, Yokoyama WM. Extending missing self? Functional interactions between lectin-like NKrp1 receptors on NK cells with lectin-like ligands. *Curr Top Microbiol Immunol* 2006;**298**:77–89.
13. Bartel Y, Bauer B, Steinle A. Modulation of NK cell function by genetically coupled C-type lectin-like receptor/ligand pairs encoded in the human natural killer gene complex. *Front Immunol* 2013;**4**:1–10.

14. Veillette A, Dong Z, Latour S. Consequence of the SLAM-SAP signaling pathway in innate-like and conventional lymphocytes. *Immunity* 2007;**27**:698–710.

15. Ma CS, Nichols KE, Tangye SG. Regulation of cellular and humoral responses by the SLAM and SAP families of molecules. *Annu Rev Immunol* 2007;**25**:337–79.

16. Chlewicki LK, Velikovsky CA, Balakrishnan V, Mariuzza RA, Kumar V. Molecular basis of the dual function of 2B4 (CD244). *J Immunol* 2008;**180**:8159–67.

17. Shibuya A, Campbell D, Hannum C, Yssel H, Franz-Bacon K, McClanahan T, et al. DNAM-1, a novel adhesion molecule involved in the cytolytic function of T lymphocytes. *Immunity* 1996;**4**:573–81.

18. Pende D, Parolini S, Pessino A, Sivori S, Augugliaro R, Morelli L, et al. Identification and molecular characterization of NKp30, a novel triggering receptor involved in natural cyto-toxicity mediated by human natural killer cells. *J Exp Med* 1999;**190**:1505–16.

19. Cantoni C, Bottino C, Vitale M, Pessino A, Augugliaro R, Malaspina A, et al. NKp44, a trig-gering receptor involved in tumor cell lysis by activated human natural killer cells, is a novel member of the immunoglobulin superfamily. *J Exp Med* 1999;**189**:787–96.

20. Sivori S, Vitale M, Morelli L, Sanseverino L, Augugliaro R, Bottino C, et al. p46, a novel natural killer cell-specific surface molecule that mediates cell activation. *J Exp Med* 1997;**186**:1129–36.

21. Spreu J, Kuttruff S, Stejfova V, Dennehy KM, Schittek B, Steinle A. Interaction of C-type lectin-like receptors NKp65 and KACL facilitates dedicated immune recognition of human keratinocytes. *Proc Natl Acad Sci U S A* 2010;**107**:5100–5.

22. Vitale M, Falco M, Castriconi R, Parolini S, Zambello R, Semenzato G, et al. Identifica-tion of NKp80, a novel triggering molecule expressed by human NK cells. *Eur J Immunol* 2001;**31**:233–42.

23. Welte S, Kuttruff S, Waldhauer I, Steinle A. Mutual activation of natural killer cells and monocytes mediated by NKp80-AICL interaction. *Nat Immunol* 2006;**7**:1334–42.

24. Lebbink RJ, de Ruiter T, Adelmeijer J, Brenkman AB, van Helvoort JM, Koch M, et al. Col-lagens are functional, high affinity ligands for the inhibitory immune receptor LAIR-1. *J Exp Med* 2006;**203**:1419–25.

25. Ito M, Maruyama T, Saito N, Koganei S, Yamamoto K, Matsumoto N. Killer cell lectin-like receptor G1 binds three members of the classical cadherin family to inhibit NK cell cytotox-icity. *J Exp Med* 2006;**203**:289–95.

26. Gründemann C, Bauer M, Schweie O, von Oppen N, Lässing U, Saudan P, et al. Cutting edge: identification of E-cadherin as a ligand for the murine killer cell lectin-like receptor G1 (KLRG1). *J Immunol* 2006;**176**:1311–5.

27. Plougastel BFM, Yokoyama WM. Immune functions encoded by the natural killer gene com-plex. *Nat Rev Immunol* 2003;**3**:304–16.

28. Anderson SK, Ortaldo JR, McVicar DW. The ever-expanding Ly49 gene family: repertoire and signaling. *Immunol Rev* 2001;**181**:79–89.

29. Lanier LL. NK cell recognition. *Annu Rev Immunol* 2005;**23**:225–74.

30. McFall E, Tu MM, Al-Khattabi N, Tai L-H, St-Laurent AS, Tzankova V, al e. Optimized tetramer analysis reveals Ly49 promiscuity for MHC ligands. *J Immunol* 2013;**191**:5722–9.

31. Franksson L, Sundbäck J, Achour A, Bernlind J, Glas R, Kärre K. Peptide dependency and selectivity of the NK inhibitory receptor Ly-49C. *Eur J Immunol* 1999;**29**:2748–58.

32. Hanke T, Takizawa H, McMahon CW, Busch DH, Pamer EG, Miller JD, et al. Direct assessment of MHC class I binding by seven Ly49 inhibitory NK cell receptors. *Immunity* 1999;**11**:67–77.

33. Deng L, Cho S, Malchiodi EL, Kerzic MC, Dam J, Mariuzza RA. Molecular architecture of the major histocompatibility complex class I-binding site of Ly49 natural killer cell recep-tors. *J Biol Chem* 2008;**283**:16840–9.

34. Dimasi N, Sawicki MW, Reineck LA, Li Y, Natarajan K, Margulies DH, et al. Crystal structure of the Ly49I natural killer cell receptor reveals variability in dimerization mode within the Ly49 family. *J Mol Biol* 2002;**320**:573–85.

35. Back J, Malchiodi EL, Cho S, Scarpellino L, Schneider P, Kerzic MC, et al. Distinct conformations of Ly49 natural killer cell receptors mediate MHC class I recognition in *trans* and *cis*. *Immunity* 2009;**31**:598–608.

36. Berry R, Ng N, Saunders PM, Vivian JP, Lin J, Deuss FA, et al. Targeting of a natural killer cell receptor family by a viral immunoevasin. *Nat Immunol* 2013;**14**:699–705.

37 Sullivan LC, Berry R, Sosnin N, Widjaja JM, Deuss FA, Balaji GR, et al. Recognition of the MHC class Ib molecule H2-Q10 by the natural killer cell receptor Ly49C. J Biol Chem 2016 pii: jbc.M116.737130.

38. Tormo J, Natarajan K, Margulies DH, Mariuzza RA. Crystal structure of a lectin-like natural killer cell receptor bound to its MHC class I ligand. *Nature* 1999;**402**:623–31.

39. Dam J, Guan R, Natarajan K, Dimasi N, Chlewicki LK, Kranz DM, et al. Variable MHC class I engagement by Ly49 NK receptors revealed by the crystal structure of Ly49C bound to H-2K^b. *Nat Immunol* 2003;**4**:1213–22.

40. Dam J, Baber J, Grishaev A, Malchiodi EL, Schuck P, Bax A, et al. Variable dimerization of the Ly49A natural killer cell receptor results in differential engagement of its MHC class I ligand. *J Mol Biol* 2006;**362**:102–13.

41. Held W, Mariuzza RA. *Cis* interactions of immunoreceptors with MHC and non-MHC ligands. *Nat Rev Immunol* 2008;**8**:269–78.

42. Held W, Mariuzza RA. Cis–trans interactions of cell surface receptors: biological roles and structural basis. *Cell Mol Life Sci* 2011;**68**:3469–78.

43. Masuda A, Nakamura A, Maeda T, Sakamoto Y, Takai T. *Cis* binding between inhibitory receptors and MHC class I can regulate mast cell activation. *J Exp Med* 2007;**204**:907–20.

44. Doucey M-A, Scarpellino L, Zimmer J, Guillaume P, Luescher IF, Bron C, et al. *Cis* association of Ly49A with MHC class I restricts natural killer cell inhibition. *Nat Immunol* 2004;**5**:328–36.

45. Back J, Chalifour A, Scarpellino L, Held W. Stable masking by H-2D^d *cis* ligand limits Ly49A relocalization to the site of NK cell/target cell contact. *Proc Natl Acad Sci U S A* 2007;**104**:3978–83.

46. Razi N, Varki A. Masking and unmasking of the sialic acid-binding lectin activity of CD22 (Siglec-2) on B lymphocytes. *Proc Natl Acad Sci U S A* 1998;**95**:7469–74.

47. Collins BE, Blixt O, AR DS, Bovin N, Marth JD, Paulson JC. Masking of CD22 by *cis* ligands does not prevent redistribution of CD22 to sites of cell contact. *Proc Natl Acad Sci U S A* 2004;**101**:6104–9.

48. Cheung TC, Oborne LM, Steinberg MW, Macauley MG, Fukuyama S, Sanjo H, et al. T cell intrinsic heterodimeric complexes between HVEM and BTLA determine receptivity to the surrounding microenvironment. *J Immunol* 2009;**183**:7286–96.

49. Haklai-Topper L, Mlechkovich G, Savariego D, Gokhman I, Yaron A. *Cis* interaction between Semaphorin6A and Plexin-A4 modulates the repulsive response to Sema6A. *EMBO J* 2010;**29**:2635–45.

50. Cordle J, Johnson S, Tay JZ, Roversi P, Wilkin MB, de Madrid BH, et al. A conserved face of the Jagged/Serrate DSL domain is involved in Notch trans-activation and cis-inhibition. *Nat Struct Mol Biol* 2008;**15**:849–57.

51. Sprinzak D, Lakhanpal A, Lebon L, Santat LA, Fontes ME, Anderson GA, et al. *Cis*-interactions between Notch and Delta generate mutually exclusive signalling states. *Nature* 2010;**465**:86–90.

52. Chalifour A, Scarpellino L, Back J, Brodin P, Devevre E, Gros F, et al. A role for *cis* interaction between the inhibitory Ly49A receptor and MHC class I for NK cell education. *Immunity* 2009;**30**:337–47.

53. Lanier LL. Evolutionary struggles between NK cells and viruses. *Nat Rev Immunol* 2008;**8**:259–68.

54. Daniels KA, Devora G, Lai WC, O'Donnell CL, Bennett M, Walsh RM. Murine cytomegalovirus is regulated by a discrete subset of natural killer cells reactive with monoclonal antibody to Ly49H. *J Exp Med* 2001;**194**:29–44.

55. Lee S-H, Girard S, Macina D, Busa M, Zafer A, Belouchi A, et al. Susceptibility to mouse cytomegalovirus is associated with depletion of an activating natural killer cell receptor of the C-type lectin superfamily. *Nat Genet* 2001;**28**:42–5.

56. Lee S-H, Zafer A, de Repentigny Y, Kothary R, Tremblay ML, Gros P, et al. Transgenic expression of the activating natural killer cell receptor Ly49H confers resistance to cytomegalovirus in genetically susceptible mice. *J Exp Med* 2003;**197**:515–26.

57. Voigt V, Forbes CA, Tonkin JN, Degli-Esposti MA, Smith HR, Yokoyama WM, et al. Murine cytomegalovirus m157 mutation and variation leads to immune evasion of natural killer cells. *Proc Natl Acad Sci U S A* 2003;**100**:13483–8.

58. French AR, Pingel JT, Wagner M, Bubic I, Yang L, Kim S, et al. Escape of mutant double-stranded DNA virus from innate immune control. *Immunity* 2004;**20**:747–56.

59. Adams EJ, Juo ZS, Venook RT, Boulanger MJ, Arase H, Lanier LL, et al. Structural elucidation of the m157 mouse cytomegalovirus ligand for Ly49 natural killer cell receptors. *Proc Natl Acad Sci U S A* 2007;**104**:10128–33.

60. Romasanta PN, Curto LM, Urtasun N, Sarratea MB, Chiappini S, Miranda MV, et al. A positive cooperativity binding model between Ly49 natural killer cell receptors and the viral immunoevasin m157: kinetic and thermodynamic studies. *J Biol Chem* 2014;**289**:5083–96.

61. Fan QR, Mosyak L, Winter CC, Wagtmann N, Long EO, Wiley DC. Structure of the inhibitory receptor for human natural killer cells resembles hematopoietic receptors. *Nature* 1997;**389**:96–100.

62. Snyder GA, Brooks AG, Sun PD. Crystal structure of the HLA-Cw3 allotype-specific killer cell inhibitory receptor KIR2DL2. *Proc Natl Acad Sci U S A* 1999;**96**:3864–9.

63. Maenaka K, Juji T, Stuart DI, Jones EY. Crystal structure of the human p58 killer cell inhibitory receptor (KIR2DL3) specific for HLA-Cw3-related MHC class I. *Structure* 1999;**7**:391–8.

64. Saulquin X, Gastinel LN, Vivier E. Crystal structure of the human natural killer cell activator receptor KIR2DS2 (CD158j). *J Exp Med* 2003;**197**:933–8.

65. Graef T, Moesta AK, Norman PJ, Abi-Rached L, Vago L, Older Aguilar AM, et al. KIR2DS4 is a product of gene conversion with KIR3DL2 that introduced specificity for HLA-A*11 while diminishing avidity for HLA-C. *J Exp Med* 2009;**206**:2557–72.

66. Boyington JC, Motyka SA, Schuck P, Brooks AG, Sun PD. Crystal structure of an NK cell immunoglobulin-like receptor in complex with its class I MHC ligand. *Nature* 2000;**405**:537–43.

67. Fan QR, Long EO, Wiley DC. Crystal structure of the human natural killer inhibitory receptor KIR2DL1-HLA-Cw4 complex. *Nat Immunol* 2001;**2**:452–60.

68. Vivian JP, Duncan RC, Berry R, O'Connor GM, Reid HH, Beddoe T, et al. Killer cell immunoglobulin-like receptor 3DL1-mediated recognition of human leukocyte antigen B. *Nature* 2011;**479**:401–5.

69. Rajakopalan S, Long EO. The direct binding of a p58 killer cell inhibitory receptor to human histocompatibility leukocyte antigen (HLA)-Cw4 exhibits peptide selectivity. *J Exp Med* 1997;**185**(1528):1523.

70. Zappacosta F, Borrego F, Brooks AG, Parker KC, Coligan JE. Peptides isolated from HLA-Cw*0304 confer different degrees of protection from natural killer cell-mediated lysis. *Proc Natl Acad Sci U S A* 1997;**94**:6313–8.

71. Alter G, Heckerman D, Schneidewind A, Fadda L, Kadie CM, Carlson JM, et al. HIV-1 adaptation to NK-cell-mediated immune pressure. *Nature* 2011;**476**:96–100.

72. Brown D, Trowsdale J, Allen R. The LILR family: modulators of innate and adaptive immune pathways in health and disease. *Tissue Antigens* 2004;**64**:215–25.

73. Cosman D, Fanger N, Borges L, Kubin M, Chin W, Peterson L, et al. A novel immunoglobulin superfamily receptor for cellular and viral MHC class I molecules. *Immunity* 1997;**7**:273–82.

74. Chapman TL, Heikema AP, West Jr. AP, Bjorkman PJ. Crystal structure and ligand binding properties of the D1D2 region of the inhibitory receptor LIR-1 (ILT-2). *Immunity* 2000;**13**:727–36.

75. Willcox BE, Thomas LM, Bjorkman PJ. Crystal structure of HLA-A2 bound to LIR-1, a host and viral major histocompatibility complex receptor. *Nat Immunol* 2003;**4**:913–9.

76. Yang Z, Bjorkman PJ. Structure of UL18, a peptide-binding viral MHC mimic, bound to a host inhibitory receptor. *Proc Natl Acad Sci U S A* 2008;**105**:10095–100.

77. Willcox BE, Thomas LM, Chapman TL, Heikema AP, West Jr. AP, Bjorkman PJ. Crystal structure of LIR-2 (ILT4) at 1.8 Å: differences from LIR-1 (ILT2) in regions implicated in the binding of the human cytomegalovirus class I MHC homolog UL18. *BMC Struct Biol* 2002;**2**:6.

78. Shiroishi M, Kuroki K, Rasubala L, Tsumoto K, Kumagai I, Kurimoto E, et al. Structural basis for recognition of the nonclassical MHC molecule HLA-G by the leukocyte Ig-like receptor B2 (LILRB2/LIR2/ILT4/CD85d). *Proc Natl Acad Sci U S A* 2006;**103**:16412–7.

79. Farrell H, Degli-Esposti M, Densley E, Cretney E, Smyth M, Davis-Poynter N. Cytomegalovirus MHC class I homologues and natural killer cells: an overview. *Microbes Infect* 2000;**2**:521–32.

80. Basta S, Bennink JR. A survival game of hide and seek: cytomegaloviruses and MHC class I antigen presentation pathways. *Viral Immunol* 2003;**16**:231–42.

81. Revilleza MJ, Wang R, Mans J, Hong M, Natarajan K, Margulies DH. How the virus outsmarts the host: function and structure of cytomegalovirus MHC-I-like molecules in the evasion of natural killer cell surveillance. *J Biomed Biotechnol* 2011;**2011**:724607.

82. Beck S, Barrell BG. Human cytomegalovirus encodes a glycoprotein homologous to MHC class I antigens. *Nature* 1988;**331**:269–72.

83. Wagner CS, Ljunggren HG, Achour A. Immune modulation by the human cytomegalovirus-encoded molecule UL18, a mystery yet to be solved. *J Immunol* 2008;**180**:19–24.

84. Fahnestock ML, Johnson JL, Feldman RM, Neveu JM, Lane WS, Bjorkman PJ. The MHC class I homolog encoded by human cytomegalovirus binds endogenous peptides. *Immunity* 1995;**3**:583–90.

85. Wagner CS, Rölle A, Cosman D, Ljunggren HG, Berndt KD, Achour A. Structural elements underlying the high binding affinity of human cytomegalovirus UL18 to leukocyte immunoglobulin-like receptor-1. *J Mol Biol* 2007;**373**:695–705.

86. Moretta A, Bottino C, Vitale M, Pende D, Cantoni C, Mingari MC, et al. Activating receptors and coreceptors involved in human natural killer cell-mediated cytolysis. *Annu Rev Immunol* 2001;**19**:197–223.

87. Moretta L, Bottino C, Pende D, Castriconi R, Mingari MC, Moretta A. Surface NK receptors and their ligands on tumor cells. *Semin Immunol* 2006;**18**:151–8.

88. Bryceson YT, Long EO. Line of attack: NK cell specificity and integration of signals. *Curr Opin Immunol* 2008;**20**:344–52.

89 Mandelboim O, Lieberman N, Lev M, Paul L, Arnon TI, Bushkin Y, et al. Recognition of haemagglutinins on virus-infected cells by NKp46 activates lysis by human NK cells. *Nature* 2001;409:1055–1060.

90. De Maria A, Fogli M, Mazza S, Basso M, Picciotto A, Costa P, et al. Increased natural cytotoxicity receptor expression and relevant IL-10 production in NK cells from chronically infected viremic HCV patients. *Eur J Immunol* 2007;**37**:445–55.

91. Hershkovitz O, Rosental B, Rosenberg LA, Navarro-Sanchez ME, Jivov S, Zilka A, et al. NKp44 receptor mediates interaction of the envelope glycoproteins from the West Nile and dengue viruses with NK cells. *J Immunol* 2009;**183**:2610–21.

92. Fuller CL, Ruthel G, Warfield KL, Swenson DL, Bosio CM, et al. NKp30-dependent cytolysis of filovirus-infected human dendritic cells. *Cell Microbiol* 2007;**9**:962–76.

93. Ho JW, Hershkovitz O, Peiris M, Zilka A, Bar-Ilan A, Nal B, et al. H5-type influenza virus hemagglutinin is functionally recognized by the natural killer-activating receptor NKp44. *J Virol* 2008;**82**:2028–32.

94. Hecht ML, Rosental B, Horlacher T, Hershkovitz O, De Paz JL, Noti C, et al. Natural cytotoxicity receptors NKp30, NKp44 and NKp46 bind to different heparan sulfate/heparin sequences. *J Proteome Res* 2009;**8**:712–20.

95. Baychelier F, Sennepin A, Ermonval M, Dorgham K, Debré P, Vieillard V. Identification of a cellular ligand for the natural cytotoxicity receptor NKp44. *Blood* 2013;**122**:2935–42.

96. Arnon TI, Achdout H, Levi O, Markel G, Saleh N, Katz G, et al. Inhibition of the NKp30 activating receptor by pp65 of human cytomegalovirus. *Nat Immunol* 2005;**6**:515–23.

97. Pogge von Strandmann E, Simhadri VR, von Tresckow B, Sasse S, Reiners KS, Hansen HP, et al. Human leukocyte antigen-B-associated transcript 3 is released from tumor cells and engages the NKp30 receptor on natural killer cells. *Immunity* 2007;**27**:965–74.

98. Brandt CS, Baratin M, Yi EC, Kennedy J, Gao Z, Fox B, et al. The B7 family member B7-H6 is a tumor cell ligand for the activating natural killer cell receptor NKp30 in humans. *J Exp Med* 2009;**206**:1495–503.

99. Zou W, Chen L. Inhibitory B7-family molecules in the tumour microenvironment. *Nat Rev Immunol* 2008;**8**:467–77.

100. Kaifu T, Escalière B, Gastinel LN, Vivier E, Baratin M. B7-H6/NKp30 interaction: a mechanism of alerting NK cells against tumors. *Cell Mol Life Sci* 2011;**68**:3531–9.

101. Cao G, Wang J, Zheng X, Wei H, Tian Z, Sun R. Tumor therapeutics work as stress inducers to enhance tumor sensitivity to natural killer (NK) cell cytolysis by up-regulating NKp30 ligand B7-H6. *J Biol Chem* 2015;**290**:29964–73.

102. Semeraro M, Rusakiewicz S, Minard-Colin V, Delahaye NF, Enot D, Vély F, et al. Clinical impact of the NKp30/B7-H6 axis in high-risk neuroblastoma patients. *Sci Transl Med* 2015;**7**:283ra55.

103. Cantoni C, Ponassi M, Biossoni R, Conte R, Spallarossa A, Moretta A, et al. The three-dimensional structure of the human NK cell receptor NKp44, a triggering partner in natural cytotoxicity. *Structure* 2003;**11**:725–34.

104. Foster CE, Colonna M, Sun PD. Crystal structure of the human natural killer (NK) cell activating receptor NKp46 reveals structural relationship to other leukocyte receptor complex immunoreceptors. *J Biol Chem* 2003;**278**:46081–6.

105. Joyce MG, Tran P, Zhuravleva MA, Jaw J, Colonna M, Sun PD. Crystal structure of human natural cytotoxicity receptor NKp30 and identification of its ligand binding site. *Proc Natl Acad Sci U S A* 2011;**108**:6223–8.

106. Li Y, Wang Q, Mariuzza RA. Structure of the human activating natural cytotoxicity receptor NKp30 bound to its tumor cell ligand B7-H6. *J Exp Med* 2011;**208**:703–14.

107. Vivier E, Tomasello E, Paul P. Lymphocyte activation via NKG2D: towards a new paradigm in immune recognition? *Curr Opin Immunol* 2002;**14**:306–11.

108. Radaev S, Rostro B, Brooks AG, Colonna M, Sun P. Conformational plasticity revealed by the co-crystal structure of the activating NK receptor NKG2D and its MHC-like ligand ULBP. *Immunity* 2001;**15**:1039–49.

109. Groh V, Steinle A, Bauer S, Spies T. Recognition of stress-induced MHC molecules by intestinal epithelial γδ T cells. *Science* 1998;**279**:1737–40.

110. Groh V, Rhinehart R, Secrist H, Bauer S, Grabstein KH, Spies T. Broad tumor-associated expression and recognition by tumor-derived γδ T cells of MICA and MICB. *Proc Natl Acad Sci U S A* 1999;**96**:6879–84.

111. Cerwenka A, Bakker AB, McClanahan T, Wagner J, Wu J, Phillips JH, et al. Retinoic acid early inducible genes define a ligand family for the activating NKG2D receptor in mice. *Immunity* 2000;**12**:721–7.

112. Diefenbach A, Jamieson AM, Liu SD, Shastri N, Raulet DH. Ligands for the murine NKG2D receptor: expression by tumor cells and activation of NK cells and macrophages. *Nat Immunol* 2000;**1**:119–26.

113. Wang R, Natarajan K, Revilleza MJ, Boyd LF, Zhi L, Zhao H, et al. Structural basis of mouse cytomegalovirus m152/gp40 interaction with RAE1γ reveals a paradigm for MHC/MHC interaction in immune evasion. *Proc Natl Acad Sci U S A* 2012;**109**:E3578–87.

114. Müller S, Zocher G, Steinle A, Stehle T. Structure of the HCMV UL16-MICB complex elucidates select binding of a viral immunoevasin to diverse NKG2D ligands. *PLoS Pathog* 2010;**6**:e1000723.

115. McFarland BJ, Kortemme T, Yu SF, Baker D, Strong RK. Symmetry recognizing asymmetry: analysis of the interactions between the C-type lectin-like immunoreceptor NKG2D and MHC class I-like ligands. *Structure* 2003;**11**:411–22.

116. Wolan DW, Teyton L, Rudolph MG, Villmow B, Bauer S, Busch DH, Wilson IA. Crystal structure of the murine NK cell-activating receptor NKG2D at 1.95 Å. *Nat Immunol* 2001;**2**:248–54.

117. Li P, Morris DL, Willcox BE, Steinle A, Spies T, Strong RK. Complex structure of the activating immunoreceptor NKG2D and its MHC class I-like ligand MICA. *Nat Immunol* 2001;**2**:443–51.

118. Li P, McDermott G, Strong RK. Crystal structure of RAE-1β and its complex with the activating immunoreceptor NKG2D. *Immunity* 2002;**16**:77–86.

119. Li P, Willie ST, Bauer S, Morris DL, Spies T, Strong RK. Crystal structure of the MHC class I homolog MICA, a γδ T cell ligand. *Immunity* 1999;**10**:577–84.

120. Lodoen M, Ogasawara K, Hamerman JA, Arase A, Houchins JP, Mocarski ES, et al. NKG2D-mediated natural killer cell protection against cytomegalovirus is impaired by viral gp40 modulation of retinoic acid early inducible 1 gene molecules. *J Exp Med* 2003;**197**:1245–53.

121. Lodoen MB, Abenes G, Umamoto S, Houchins JP, Liu F, Lanier LL. The cytomegalovirus m155 gene product subverts natural killer cell antiviral protection by disruption of H60-NKG2D interactions. *J Exp Med* 2004;**200**:1075–81.

122. Krmpotic A, Hasan M, Loewendorf A, Saulig T, Halenius A, Lenac T, et al. NK cell activation through the NKG2D ligand MULT-1 is selectively prevented by mouse cytomegalovirus gene m145. *J Exp Med* 2005;**201**:211–20.

123. Borrego F, Ulbrecht M, Weiss EH, Coligan JE, Brooks AG. Recognition of human histocompatibility leukocyte antigen (HLA)-E complexed with HLA class I signal sequence-derived peptides by CD94/NKG2 confers protection from natural killer cell-mediated lysis. *J Exp Med* 1998;**187**:813–8.

124. Braud VM, Allan DS, O'Callaghan CA, Söderström K, D'Andrea A, Ogg GS, et al. HLA-E binds to natural killer cell receptors CD94/NKG2A, B and C. *Nature* 1998;**391**:795–9.

125. Lee N, Llano M, Carretero M, Ishitani A, Navarro F, López-Botet M, et al. HLA-E is a major ligand for the natural killer inhibitory receptor CD94/NKG2A. *Proc Natl Acad Sci U S A* 1998;**95**:5199–204.

126. Sullivan LC, Clements CS, Beddoe T, Johnson D, Hoare HL, Lin J, Huyton T, et al. The heterodimeric assembly of the CD94-NKG2 receptor family and implications for human leukocyte antigen-E recognition. *J Exp Med* 2008;**205**:725–35.

127. Petrie EJ, Clements CS, Lin J, Sullivan LC, Johnson D, Huyton T, et al. CD94-NKG2A recognition of human leukocyte antigen (HLA)-E bound to an HLA class I leader sequence. *J Exp Med* 2008;**205**:725–35.

128. Kaiser BK, Pizarro JC, Kerns J, Strong RK. Structural basis for NKG2A/CD94 recognition of HLA-E. *Proc Natl Acad Sci U S A* 2008;**105**:6696–701.

129. Guthman MD, Tal M, Pecht I. A secretion inhibitory signal transduction molecule on mast cells is another C-type lectin. *Proc Natl Acad Sci U S A* 1995;**92**:9397–401.

130. Hanke T, Corral L, Vance RE, Raulet DH. 2F1 antigen, the mouse homolog of the rat "mast cell function-associated antigen", is a lectin-like type II transmembrane receptor expressed by natural killer cells. *Eur J Immunol* 1998;**28**:4409–17.

131. Voehringer D, Blaser P, Brawand P, Raulet DH, Hanke T, Pircher H. Viral infections induce adundant numbers of senescent CD8 T cells. *J Immunol* 2001;**167**:4838–43.

132. Robbins SH, Terrizzi SC, Sydora BC, Mikayama T, Brossay L. Differential regulation of killer cell lectin-like receptor G1 expression on T cells. *J Immunol* 2003;**170**:5876–85.

133. Thimme R, Appay V, Koschella M, Panther E, Roth E, Hislop AD, et al. Increased expression of the NK cell receptor KLRG1 by virus-specific CD8 T cells during persistent antigen stimulation. *J Virol* 2005;**79**:12112–6.

134. Ibegbu CC, Xu YX, Harris W, Maggio D, Miller JD, Koutis AP. Expression of killer cell lectin-like receptor G1 on antigen-specific human CD8$^+$ T lymphocytes during active, latent, and resolved infection and its relation with CD57. *J Immunol* 2005;**174**:6088–94.

135. Tessmer MS, Fugere C, Stevenaert F, Naidenko OV, Chong HJ, Leclercq G, et al. KLRG1 binds cadherins and preferentially associates with SHIP-1. *Int Immunol* 2007;(4)391–400.

136. Gumbiner BM. Regulation of cadherin-mediated adhesion in morphogenesis. *Nat Rev Mol Cell Biol* 2005;**6**:622–34.

137. Colonna M. Cytolytic responses: cadherins put out the fire. *J Exp Med* 2006;**203**:261–4.

138. Schwartzkopff S, Gründemann C, Schweier O, Rosshart S, Karjalainen KE, Becker K-F, et al. Tumor-associated E-cadherin mutations affect binding to the killer cell lectin-like receptor G1 in humans. *J Immunol* 2007;**179**:1022–9.

139. Jeanes A, Gottardi CJ, Yap AS. Cadherins and cancer: how does cadherin dysfunction promote tumor progression? *Oncogene* 2008;**24**:6920–9.

140. Li Y, Hofmann M, Wang Q, Teng L, Chlewicki LK, Pircher H, et al. Structure of natural killer cell receptor KLRG1 bound to E-cadherin reveals basis for MHC-independent missing self recognition. *Immunity* 2009;**31**:35–46.

141. Hao L, Klein J, Nei M. Heterogeneous but conserved natural killer receptor gene complexes in four major orders of mammals. *Proc Natl Acad Sci U S A* 2006;**103**:3192–7.

142. Iizuka K, Naidenko OV, Plougastel BF, Fremont DH, Yokoyama WM. Genetically linked C-type lectin-related ligands for the NKRP1 family of natural killer cell receptors. *Nat Immunol* 2003;**4**:801–7.

143. Carlyle JR, Jamieson AM, Gasser S, Clingan CS, Arase H, Raulet DH. Missing self recognition of Ocil/Clr-b by inhibitory NKR-P1 natural killer cell receptors. *Proc Natl Acad Sci U S A* 2004;**101**:3527–32.

144. Aldemir H, Prod'homme V, Dumaurier MJ, Retiere C, Poupon G, Cazareth J, et al. Cutting edge: lectin-like transcript 1 is a ligand for the CD161 receptor. *J Immunol* 2005;**175**:7791–5.

145. Rosen DB, Bettadapura J, Alsharifi M, Mathew PA, Warren HS, Lanier LL. Cutting edge: lectin-like transcript-1 is a ligand for the inhibitory human NKR-P1A receptor. *J Immunol* 2005;**175**:7796–9.

146. Rosen DB, Cao W, Avery DT, Tangye SG, Liu YJ, Houchins JP, et al. Functional consequences of interactions between human NKR-P1A and its ligand LLT1 expressed on activated dendritic cells and B cells. *J Immunol* 2008;**180**:6508–17.

147. Germain C, Meier A, Jensen T, Knapnougel P, Poupon G, Lazzari A, et al. Induction of lectin-like transcript 1 (LLT1) protein cell surface expression by pathogens and interferon-γ contributes to modulate immune responses. *J Biol Chem* 2011;**286**:37964–75.

148. Klimosch SN, Bartel Y, Wiemann S, Steinle A. Genetically coupled receptor-ligand pair NKp80-AICL enables autonomous control of human NK cell responses. *Blood* 2013;**122**:2380–99.

149. Vogler I, Steinle A. Vis-à-vis in the NKC: genetically linked natural killer cell receptor/ligand pairs in the natural killer gene complex (NKC). *J Innate Immun* 2011;**3**:227–35.

150. Skálová T, Kotýnková K, Dušková J, Hašek J, Koval T, Kolenko P, et al. Mouse Clr-g, a ligand for NK cell activation receptor NKR-P1F: crystal structure and biophysical properties. *J Immunol* 2012;**189**:4881–9.

151. Kolenko P, Rozbeský D, Vaněk O, Jr KV, Hofbauerová K, Novák P, et al. Molecular architecture of mouse activating NKR-P1 receptors. *J Struct Biol* 2011;**175**:434–41.

152. Kita S, Matsubara H, Kasai Y, Tamaoki T, Okabe Y, Fukuhara H, et al. Crystal structure of extracellular domain of human lectin-like transcript 1 (LLT1), the ligand for natural killer receptor-P1A. *Eur J Immunol* 2015;**45**:1605–13.

153. Li Y, Wang Q, Chen S, Brown PH, Mariuzza RA. Structure of NKp65 bound to its keratinocyte ligand reveals basis for genetically linked recognition in natural killer gene complex. *Proc Natl Acad Sci U S A* 2013;**110**:11505–10.

Chapter 5

Structure-Function in Antibodies to Double-Stranded DNA

Yumin Xia*, Ertan Eryilmaz*, David Cowburn*, Chaim Putterman[†]
*Albert Einstein College of Medicine, New York, NY, United States, [†]Albert Einstein College of Medicine and Montefiore Medical Center, Bronx, NY, United States

5.1 ANTI-dsDNA ANTIBODIES ARE PIVOTAL IN THE PATHOGENESIS OF LUPUS ERYTHEMATOSUS

Systemic lupus erythematosus (SLE) is a multifactorial autoimmune disease affecting multiple organs. Despite variable clinical manifestations of differing severity, patients with SLE have in common high titers of serum autoantibodies that target normal tissues or cells. The binding to self-antigens or formation of immune complexes can subsequently trigger pronounced inflammatory responses, which lead to further injury and subsequently functional deficits in target organs. Although almost all tissues and organs can be affected in patients with SLE, the kidneys, skin, brain, and joints are most frequently involved. Renal involvement, also known as lupus nephritis, is found in up to 60% of adults with SLE[1] and is among the three most common causes of death (together with infection and circulatory system diseases) in lupus patients.[2–5]

Several complications in SLE are closely associated with the robust autoantibody production that characterizes this disease. To date, 180 types of autoantibodies have been detected in lupus sera.[6] These autoantibodies, a subset of which are actually pathogenic, may recognize components of nuclei, cytoplasm, and membranes, plasma or extracellular matrix proteins, and other tissue antigens.[6] Similar autoantibodies can also be seen in the lupus-prone mouse models (e.g., MRL-lpr/lpr, NZB×NBW F1).[7] Indeed, among all recognized autoimmune diseases, SLE has the largest number of serum autoantibodies associated with it. The heterogeneity of clinical manifestations in SLE perhaps reflects the complexity of the pathogenic autoantibody response in this disease.

Of the SLE-related autoantibodies, double-stranded DNA (dsDNA) antibodies have received the most intense experimental attention. These antibodies are highly specific for SLE and are believed to play an instrumental role in lupus glomerulonephritis[8] (more on that later), and most likely in skin and

Structural Biology in Immunology. https://doi.org/10.1016/B978-0-12-803369-2.00005-X

brain disease as well. Recently, highlighting the recognized association between anti-DNA antibodies and lupus nephritis, the Systemic Lupus International Collaborating Clinics (SLICC) consortium proposed a new diagnostic scheme (so-called SLICC-12) for the classification of SLE. An important change over the previous widely used ACR criteria was that biopsy-proven lupus nephritis in combination with the presence of anti-dsDNA antibodies is sufficient to make a diagnosis of SLE, even in the absence of other characteristic organ manifestations.[9]

As mentioned earlier, anti-dsDNA antibodies are not only a serological hallmark of SLE but also critical in the pathogenesis of lupus nephritis. In mice, anti-dsDNA antibodies can be eluted from kidneys harvested from lupus nephritis models[10] and were significantly highly enriched as compared to serum. To investigate the capacity of anti-dsDNA antibodies to produce glomerular immune deposits and nephritis, normal mice were administered with monoclonal anti-dsDNA antibodies derived from different lupus-prone models.[11] These anti-dsDNA IgGs deposited in glomeruli, and in normal mice induced proteinuria and histological changes similar to lupus nephritis. Furthermore, non-autoimmune mice made transgenic for an anti-dsDNA immunoglobulin heavy chain developed lupus-like nephritis.[12]

Clinical evidence also indicates a close association between anti-dsDNA antibodies and renal injury in patients with SLE. A surge in anti-dsDNA antibody titers predicts the subsequent development of a severe SLE flare within 6 months.[13] Corticosteroid therapy can prevent subsequent severe disease flares in patients with serologically active but clinically inactive SLE, through decreasing the serum titers of anti-dsDNA antibodies.[14] Consequently, targeting high anti-DNA antibody titers for reduction may represent a valuable strategy for the treatment of lupus nephritis.[15] Thus, although renal disease can occur in murine models and human patients also in their absence, there is convincing experimental and clinical evidence that anti-dsDNA antibodies are often associated with, and play a role in, the development of lupus nephritis.

There are multiple ways by which anti-dsDNA antibodies may contribute to the pathogenesis of renal injury in SLE. Anti-dsDNA antibodies can indirectly and directly cross-react with glomerular components including resident cells, intracellular components, and extracellular matrix such as the glomerular basement membrane.[16–21] In addition, anti-dsDNA antibodies can penetrate into living cells such as macrophages and mesangial cells.[22,23] Moreover, anti-dsDNA IgG upregulates the gene expression of proinflammatory cytokines in murine mesangial cells via binding to high-mobility group-binding protein 1, leading to kidney cell proliferation.[24] Furthermore, IgG anti-dsDNA antibodies isolated from lupus sera can induce myofibroblast-like morphological features in mesangial cells, a phenotype which is one of the histological characteristics of lupus glomeruli.[25,26] Therefore, through several possible types of interactions with self-antigens in the kidneys, anti-dsDNA antibodies can contribute to renal injury.

5.2 THE BASIC FEATURES OF ANTIGEN RECOGNITION BY ANTI-dsDNA ANTIBODIES

DNA as an antigen possesses unique features because of the variability inherent in the structure of this highly charged polymer.[27] This heterogeneity, in DNA origin, size, conformation, and mobility, can affect its antigenicity. Moreover, DNA may bind to anti-dsDNA antibodies through monovalent or bivalent interactions, based on its extended polynucleotide structure.[27] For the most part, DNA autoantibody recognition of DNA depends on the interaction between helical protein segments and bases in the major DNA groove, and contacts of other antibody segments with both the phosphate backbone and minor groove.[28] Therefore, the structure of DNA (or DNA-mimicking antigens) can affect their interaction with anti-dsDNA antibodies. Furthermore, deeper appreciation of the nature of DNA as an antigen may help in the interpretation of tests used clinically for diagnostic purposes and improve their standardization.

Modification of DNA can improve antigenicity under certain conditions. For example, hydroxyl radical modified-DNA induces antibodies that have antigen-binding properties similar to naturally occurring anti-DNA autoantibodies.[29] Anti-dsDNA antibodies also show specific binding to Z-DNA, which is formed in vitro and whose conformation is stabilized by a Z-DNA-binding protein.[30] The length of linear DNA may affect the binding strength of anti-dsDNA antibodies with DNA antigens. To date, the shortest DNA molecule found to interact with DNA-binding antibodies is an 18 bp single-stranded DNA fragment, which exhibits antigenic properties similar to dsDNA when it binds to anti-DNA antibodies.[28,31] It was found that IgG anti-dsDNA antibodies bind to the $(dG-dC)_3$ and $(dG-dC)_4$ cores in double-stranded octadecanucleotides.[28] To investigate if anti-DNA antibodies might prefer to interact with damaged or modified DNA over the native form,[32] the crystal structure of a complex of native dsDNA bound to the Fab fragment of an anti-dsDNA antibody was compared to that of a modified complex created in silico, in which the dsDNA was altered to contain a dimerized thymine (as can result from photo damage of DNA). Both complexes were then subjected to molecular dynamics simulations, and the in silico equilibrium properties of the Fab fragments were compared. Interestingly, it was found that the Fab fragment binds to the modified (damaged) dsDNA with higher affinity, forming a stronger immune complex.[32]

Anti-dsDNA antibodies are notable for cross-reacting with non-DNA antigens. Anti-dsDNA antibodies can not only bind to DNA fragments of different sizes but also recognize single-stranded (ss)DNA and even RNA molecules. Affinity-purified anti-dsDNA IgG and monoclonal anti-dsDNA antibodies immunoprecipitate 18S ribosomal RNA from DNase-treated cell extracts.[33] Immunization of rabbits with complexes of RNA with methylated bovine serum albumin stimulates production of IgG antibodies that recognize DNA and RNA and exhibit RNase and DNase activities.[34] Moreover, as noted earlier, anti-dsDNA antibodies can bind to a broad spectrum of non-nucleic acid self-antigens, including resident cells (e.g., mesangial cells, glomerular endothelial cells, podocytes, keratinocytes, HEp-2 cells), cellular components (e.g., histones, cardiolipin, alpha-actinin, annexin II, C1q), and extracellular matrix (including laminin, matrigel, collagen II, collagen IV, and fibronectin).[16–21,35–40] Moreover, anti-dsDNA antibodies cross-react with a phage library displaying 8–15 amino acid long peptides.[41–46] Such cross-reaction between anti-dsDNA antibodies and multiple self-antigens that derive from renal and other tissues may contribute to both tissue specificity and pathogenicity, but may also offer a possible avenue for the development of novel inhibitors of antibody binding to tissue.

5.3 THE CONSTANT REGIONS CONTRIBUTE TO ANTIGENIC SPECIFICITY AND RENAL PATHOGENICITY OF ANTI-dsDNA ANTIBODIES

According to the classic view, the variable regions are the part of the antibody structure that exclusively determines antibody binding. However, recent studies have conclusively demonstrated that constant regions also contribute to antibody affinity and specificity.[47,48] In several antibody systems, isotype switching leads to altered binding of antibodies. For example, the variable region identical IgA and IgE antibodies to Cryptococcus neoformans capsular polysaccharide manifest specificity differences.[49] Much more on the relevant studies regarding the protective antibody response can be found in the contribution by Bowen and Casedavall elsewhere in this volume.

In the case of anti-dsDNA antibodies, in both animal models and human disease, certain isotypes exhibit a tighter link with the induction of renal injury. In lupus patients, serum IgG1 anti-dsDNA antibody titers frequently rise prior to the clinical expression (flare) of glomerulonephritis.[50] To identify a possible relationship between specific constant regions and end-organ damage, the serum distribution and renal deposition of specific anti-dsDNA IgG subclasses were analyzed over time as a function of disease activity in patients with SLE.[50] IgG1 anti-dsDNA antibodies increased in almost all patients prior to a renal relapse, but only in less than half the patients with an extra-renal relapse. In lupus-prone mice (MRL/lpr, BXSB, and NZB × NZW F1), glomerular eluates contained a restricted number of DNA-binding antibodies in a pH range of 8.0–9.0.[51] The murine IgG3 isotype has the property of forming self-associating complexes and generating cryoglobulins. Therefore, rheumatoid factors and anti-dsDNA autoantibodies of the IgG3 isotype may have greater potential to induce lupus nephritis.[52] Finally, the TH_1 cytokine interferon-gamma can promote class-switching to the IgG2a and IgG3 isotypes. Indeed, TH_1-driven autoimmune responses are vital in the generation of highly pathogenic lupus autoantibodies.[52]

To directly examine if the isotype of anti-dsDNA antibodies affects renal pathogenicity, a panel of five anti-dsDNA antibodies which share identical variable regions, representing each of the murine immunoglobulin subclasses (IgM, IgG1, IgG2b, IgG2a, and IgG3), was generated.[53] In vitro, the IgG2a and IgG3 isotypes had higher affinity for renal self-antigens, which was reflected in vivo in increased IgG deposition in kidneys and worse renal damage in SCID mice injected with hybridoma cells of these IgG2a and IgG3 anti-dsDNA clones. These results suggest that the constant region materially contributes to the nephritogenicity of anti-dsDNA antibodies, through enhancing immunoglobulin affinity and modulating fine specificity.

5.4   THE STRUCTURE OF ANTI-dsDNA ANTIBODIES

Since constant regions have an essential role in determining the pathogenic potential of anti-dsDNA antibodies, it would be instructive to elucidate the mechanisms by which the constant regions affect the binding of anti-dsDNA antibodies to self-antigens. Three isotype-switch variants (IgG1, IgG2a, and IgG2b) were generated from an IgG3 isotype of the PL9–11 murine anti-dsDNA antibody[54] (all isotypes share identical variable regions in both light and heavy chains). By surface plasmon resonance, significant differences were found in histone-binding affinity between members of this panel of anti-dsDNA antibodies. Tryptophan fluorescence can determine a wavelength shift upon antibody binding to antigen. The shifts in emission wavelength of tryptophan fluorescence were dependent on the isotype of anti-dsDNA antibodies as they bound to DNA and histone. Moreover, circular dichroism spectroscopy quantitatively measured the changes in secondary structure contents (including turns, regular α helix, regular β strand, distorted α helix, distorted β strand, and unordered) that differed between isotypes upon antigen binding. Therefore, the effects of antigen binding of antibodies were also constant region dependent. We should note that the secondary structural alterations affected by constant regions may also provide a convincing explanation for the differences in the fine specificity observed between anti-dsDNA antibodies with similarities in their variable regions, as well as the frequent cross-reactions observed between anti-dsDNA antibodies and non-nuclear antigens.[54]

These results in a unique anti-DNA antibody model system are consistent with previous reports demonstrating that both antigen recognition and affinity of antibodies are molecular features that may not be solely dictated by the variable regions.[20,55–58] Furthermore, changes in the secondary structure that occur in antibodies upon binding to antigens may vary, depending on antibody subclass.[59] Finally, the constant region can confer new properties to immunoglobulin molecules, in their proteolytic capacity and electronic emission spectra.[59] Thus, constant regions may directly influence antibody-antigen interactions through alteration of antibody structure in both protective and pathogenic antibody responses.

Another interesting observation was that the tryptophan fluorescence of anti-dsDNA antibodies can be affected by changing ionic strength.[54] In titration experiments, increasing NaCl concentrations can induce tighter antigen-antibody binding, thus further burying tryptophans and excluding solvent molecules. Consequently, the polarity of the interaction decreases, resulting in shifts in fluorescence emission wavelengths. By surface plasmon resonance, the binding affinity of an anti-dsDNA antibody (IgG2a isotype) to histones had an inverse correlation with salt concentrations. The explanation we proposed for this phenomenon was that at least part of the interaction between anti-dsDNA antibodies and self-antigens is electrostatic, and therefore NaCl can compete with antibody in the binding to histone and consequently alter tryptophan fluorescence. The conclusion from these experiments is that the constant regions apparently affect the binding of anti-dsDNA antibodies to DNA (as well as other antigens) by changing local electronic environments and the secondary structures of these antibodies.

Structural analysis of anti-dsDNA antibodies can provide critical clues to the molecular mechanisms underlying both their antigenic specificity and renal pathogenicity. The binding specificity of an antibody is dictated by six loops, three on each V_H and $V_{Kappa/Lambda}$ regions. These loops are called complementarity-determining regions (CDRs). They engage and can collectively bind to the specific antigen. In an immature antibody, both CDRs and framework residues are identical to their germline sequences. As antibodies go through maturation in germinal centers, the amino-acid compositions of CDRs change through a process called somatic hypermutation. After this maturation process, any number of CDR loops can make up the paratopes (also known as the antigen binding region—the part of the antibody which actually binds the antigen). Those CDR loops/amino acids which are not involved in antigen binding are usually identical to their germline versions.[59] The NZB lupus-prone strain that rarely develops nephritis has several highly homologous germ-line V_H genes that encode less cationic anti-dsDNA antibodies,[60] indicating that the charge in variable regions may sometimes be relevant to pathogenicity.

The structural basis of autoantibody binding to DNA and the renal pathogenicity of this antibody class is not fully understood. Therefore, direct three-dimensional structural information concerning autoantibody-DNA complexes can provide valuable insight. While crystallization of whole IgG molecules with DNA has not been successful to date, the study of Fab or F(ab')$_2$ fragments of anti-DNA IgGs, alone or antigen bound, was achievable. To understand the interactions between anti-DNA antibodies and DNA antigen, the crystal structure of a complex of a recombinant Fab (DNA-1) with a dT5 oligo was analyzed.[61] The DNA-1 clone was isolated from a lupus prone strain using a bacteriophage Fab display library. The crystal structure indicated that DNA-1 binds to the oligo through the intertwining of the thymine bases between its tyrosine side chains, which facilitates sequence-specific hydrogen bond formation with the thymines' bases. Specific tyrosine residues of particular importance in this reaction were light chain 32, 49, 100, and heavy chain 100A, with contribution of hydrogen bonds by other residues.

This study further suggested that arginine side chains in the heavy chain CDR3 play an important role in antibody-DNA binding, through maintaining the structural integrity of the antigen-binding domain rather than forming salt bridges. The contribution of arginine residues to DNA specificity has been confirmed by other studies. A52 is a murine monoclonal IgG anti-DNA antibody isolated from a lupus prone NZB × NZW F1 mouse.[62] The analysis of the A52 Fab fragment showed that the CDR3 of the heavy chain contains four arginine residues in close proximity, which provide a strong positive charge and in this fashion creating an accommodating surface for DNA antigen to bind. By reverting the heavy and light chain sequences to their germline configuration and performing site-directed mutagenesis of arginine residues in the CDR3 region of the 412.67 anti-DNA antibody, it was found that arginines at both position 105 and 107 exhibit solvent-exposed orientation at the peak of the main loop of this CDR3 region and therefore facilitate DNA binding. While both arginines were mandatory for binding to dsDNA, one arginine alone, at position 105 or 107, was adequate to confer specificity for ssDNA.[63] These results were consistent with other reports that anti-DNA antibody pathogenicity is correlated to the arginine content in the antibody.[23,64] Besides arginine, asparagine, and lysine residues in anti-DNA CDRs also facilitate DNA binding.[65] These findings are in fact not surprising; as DNA is a negatively charged molecule, charge complementarity within the paratopes of DNA-binding antibodies would be predicted to be important. Arginine and lysine are basic amino acids and can create the positively charged complementary surfaces for DNA binding. Polar amino acids, such as Asn, Gln, Ser, and Thr, can form hydrogen bonds and hence stabilize interactions.

However, charge is by no means the sole or most important determinant of antigen binding by anti-DNA antibodies. Careful analysis of anti-dsDNA antibodies with closely related variable region sequences and differing pathogenic properties would illuminate the contribution of specific motifs to pathogenicity.[66] The approach we used to address this question was to create a panel of mutants of the murine IgG anti-dsDNA 99D.7E antibody with targeted substitutions of particular amino acid residues in the heavy chain. Contrary to what might be expected, we found that neither charge nor dsDNA affinity was sufficient for prediction of the pathogenicity of (certain) anti-dsDNA antibodies.[67] Moreover, differences in fine specificity induced by single mutations, rather than differences in dsDNA affinity, drastically affected the nephritogenic potential (site of immunoglobulin deposition) of anti-dsDNA antibodies.

Antibody binding may also shift the folding equilibrium of DNA. The 5′-d [CTG(CCTT)CAG]-3′ oligo sequence was predicted to form a hairpin, consisting of a CCTT loop and a three base-pair stem. However, when cocrystallized with the DNA-1 anti-dsDNA Fab, the bound antigen had a conformation that differed prominently from the predicted conformation.[68] Moreover, the Fab binds preferentially to the unstructured state of the DNA antigen.

Continuing efforts in ever more detailed structural analysis of anti-dsDNA antibodies may contribute to elucidating their role in specific tissue injury in SLE. Structural differences likely underlie the diverse pathogenic potential of anti-dsDNA antibodies, which may not only explain why specific isotypes are associated with particular disease characteristics and manifestations but also help in the design of antibodies for therapeutic purposes.

5.5 CATALYTIC PROPERTIES OF ANTI-dsDNA ANTIBODIES

A catalytic antibody, also called an abzyme or catmab, is an antibody harboring catalytic potential.[69] While antibodies with catalytic activity can be generated in the laboratory, abzymes are also found in healthy individuals and in patients with lupus and other autoimmune diseases, where they may recognize and then hydrolyze DNA antigens.[70,71] Moreover, naturally occurring catalytic antibodies can be found in patients with viral and bacterial infections.[72] It has been proposed that catalytic antibodies may have important functional roles in homeostasis, autoimmune diseases, and in protection against infection. Enzymes function via catalysis of the transition between reactants and final products in a chemical reaction by reducing the activation energy required. Similarly, antibodies may be designed for stabilizing otherwise unstable intermediate reactants, and as a result catalyze these chemical reactions.[73] With its potential uses for biotechnological purposes, the discovery of catalytic antibodies has been very exciting—potentially opening up new opportunities and applications in the scientific realms of enzymology, immunology, and chemistry.

DNA-catalyzing antibodies were first described by Shuster et al.[74] These antibodies resist acid shock and degrade DNA in patterns distinct from those seen with DNase enzymes. Since then, additional studies have pointed to the potential importance of DNA-catalyzing antibodies in the pathogenesis of SLE, with increased concentrations of dsDNA-hydrolyzing autoantibodies described in the sera of both lupus mice and human disease.[75,76,78] Anti-DNA antibodies with catalytic potential have in common with the enzyme DNase I several identical or similar amino acid residues which are necessary for binding of calcium and magnesium, as well as for DNA hydrolysis.[77] Catalytic anti-DNA antibodies might be targeted to enter the nuclei of neoplastic cells and even actually kill these tumoral cells through DNA hydrolysis.[78]

It is, however, important to point out that while catalytic antibodies can kill cells in vitro, whether this happens in vivo or whether this phenomenon can be utilized therapeutically is far from settled. For secreted antibodies to get to the nucleus in a living cell, they have to be internalized, not recycled back to outside the cell, pass through the reducing environment in the cytoplasm without losing function, and then pass through the nucleopores. Therefore, for enough antibodies to reach the nucleus for any therapeutic effect, it is likely that very high doses would be needed because only a fraction of the antibodies injected may reach the intended target. Accordingly, a catalytic/cytotoxic effect seen in vitro may not immediately be potentially translatable into a therapeutic application.

We had demonstrated that murine anti-dsDNA antibodies can exhibit antigenic cross-reactivity and renal pathogenicity which were subclass dependent.[20] Using the same panel of murine IgG anti-dsDNA antibodies described earlier that share identical variable regions but different constant regions (PL9–11 derived), Xia et al. found that these isotypes vary significantly in catalytic cleavage of both ssDNA and dsDNA.[31] Furthermore, these anti-dsDNA antibodies not only cleave DNA but also hydrolyze a 12-mer peptide (ALWPPNLHAWVP, abbreviated as "ALW"), which binds to anti-dsDNA antibodies specifically.[41] Moreover, anti-dsDNA antibodies cleave both DNA and the ALW peptide in a reaction which was both time- and temperature dependent. Interestingly, although the various anti-dsDNA isotypes (IgG1, IgG2a, IgG2b, IgG3) were found to initially attack the ALW peptide at the same sites in the sequence, the binding affinity of the antibodies to ALW did not correlate with proteolysis rates. These results indicate that the catalytic properties of anti-dsDNA antibodies are isotype dependent. Another conclusion would be that when designing antibodies for clinical use, one also needs to consider whatever catalytic properties may be conferred by the antibody constant region.[31]

The presence of a catalytic antibody can be detected based on its catalytic properties. Therefore, there are no unique methods to identify catalytic antibodies because the antigens may be protein, DNA or RNA, molecules which obviously differ from each other widely in chemical properties and structure, and the substrates may be entirely different from the antigen. Specifically, DNA-binding antibodies can be assessed for DNase catalytic potential by agarose gel electrophoresis[31] or microtiter plate assay.[79] The affinity-linked oligonucleotide nuclease assay (ALONA) is another approach for detection of abzyme potential, in which the oligo has a 3′-biotinylated DNA strand (substrate) labeled at 5′-end with digoxigenin. This substrate can then bind specifically to streptavidin-coated microtiter wells; following binding of the antibody of interest, uncleaved substrate that retains its digoxigenin tag can be easily detected with the appropriate specific antibody. The ALONA procedure can be applied to high-throughput screening, for example, for studying a large number of hybridoma clones derived from murine lupus models. For peptide catalysis, mass spectrometry can be used to identify the sequences of peptide fragments after incubation of antibodies with targeted peptides.[31] Moreover, nuclear magnetic resonance (NMR) may assign the backbone resonances of the isotope labeled peptides that are bound by anti-dsDNA antibodies.[31]

Since peptides that mimic the antigenicity of DNA can block the cross-reaction of lupus anti-dsDNA antibodies with glomerular antigens, these represent a potentially useful approach for inhibiting the nephritogenicity of autoantibodies with this specificity.[41] However, proteolysis of these peptides by catalytic anti-dsDNA antibodies may limit their utility. Identifying the specific sites and amino acid sequences which are being targeted by the antibody for cleavage may be important; with this knowledge, the appropriate structural changes can be introduced so that the peptides would become less susceptible to hydrolysis in vivo.[31] The ALW peptide had the same first-attack sites for all the tested anti-dsDNA isotypes and therefore would potentially be a good candidate to be chemically modified or transformed to a peptidomimetic to serve as an inhibitor of the in vivo interactions between autoantibodies and self-antigen.[31]

5.6 DNA-MIMICKING PEPTIDES BOUND BY ANTI-dsDNA ANTIBODIES

Developing specific inhibitors of pathogenic anti-dsDNA antibodies has been challenging. Nevertheless, since peptides can mimic the antigenicity of DNA, they conceivably may block the binding of anti-dsDNA antibodies to self-antigens through competing with DNA for binding sites. Therefore, peptide DNA mimics might prevent the deposition of anti-dsDNA antibodies in kidneys (and/or other organs) and the ensuing tissue damage. Several peptides have been shown to display such properties.

The hypothesis that peptide epitopes may mimic a DNA structure was first demonstrated by in vitro experiments. R4A is a murine anti-dsDNA antibody of the IgG2b isotype that deposits in kidney glomeruli and induces histological injury following in vivo administration.[80] Using peptide display phage libraries, several peptides were identified that specifically reacted with R4A.[81] These peptides bound preferentially to R4A when compared with two closely related antibodies (95 and 52b3) generated by site-directed mutagenesis, yet which differed significantly from the parent R4A in nephritogenic potential.[80] Further support that a peptide can serve as a molecular DNA mimic could be found in studies in which administration of the D-form of the R4A-specific peptide (DWEYS) protected mice from the renal deposition of the R4A antibody.[80]

If peptides isolated via phage library technology can display mimotope activity (i.e., mimicking the epitope structure), they would provoke an antibody response similar to that stimulated by the original epitope. To determine whether peptide DNA surrogates may trigger antinuclear autoimmune responses, BALB/c mice were immunized with the DWEYSVWLSN peptide in a multimerized form. Surprisingly, about 3 weeks after their initial immunization, this originally non-autoimmune mouse strain began to develop high titers of IgG anti-dsDNA antibodies.[84] Immunized mice also produced antibodies to other autoantigens and displayed renal IgG deposition. Indeed, these peptide-elicited anti-dsDNA antibodies were structurally similar to spontaneously appearing autoantibodies in lupus-prone mice.[82] Therefore, immunization with phage display isolated peptide can stimulate a pathogenic lupus-like anti-dsDNA response in non-autoimmune mice. In a similar type of experiment, three monoclonal IgG2a anti-dsDNA antibodies were derived from lupus-prone mice of the NZB × NZW

F1 strain.[83] Peptides selected by these antibodies could bind to serum antibodies from human patients with SLE. Moreover, BALB/c mice immunized with these peptides displayed increased IgG3 anti-dsDNA antibodies in the serum.[83] Hence, besides contributing to our understanding of the epitope spreading that occurs in lupus, these peptide-induced autoimmunity models can also help identify potential blocking antigens that might be therapeutic. Peptide-based passive immunotherapies, by virtue of their focus on blocking antibody binding to target organs and thus preventing subsequent injury (rather than by non-specific immunosuppression which also interferes with protective immunity), may be emerging as a novel therapeutic approach in the treatment of lupus.

Similar experiments were done with human lupus autoantibodies.[87] Affinity-purified polyclonal human anti-dsDNA IgGs were found to specifically bind a 15-mer peptide, ASPVTARVLWKASHV. ASPVTARVLWKASHV bound to anti-dsDNA antibodies in ELISA and dot blot assays and inhibited anti-dsDNA antibody binding.[87]

As mentioned earlier, ALW is a 12-mer peptide selected by a panel of murine anti-DNA IgGs (PL9–11 IgG1, IgG2a, IgG2b, and IgG3) that share identical variable regions.[41] The binding of PL9–11 IgGs to antigens including DNA, laminin, kidney cells, and rat glomeruli was significantly reduced upon the preincubation with ALW. Moreover, by alanine scanning, we confirmed that the binding of ALW to anti-DNA antibodies was amino acid sequence specific. Interestingly, the binding of lupus sera from both murine models and human patients to dsDNA and, importantly, to glomerular antigens, was significantly inhibited by the ALW peptide. The DNA-mimicking peptides reported previously were selected by a single isotype or lupus sera, while the ALW peptide binds to all four IgG isotypes and should then more broadly inhibit the pathogenic polyclonal anti-DNA antibody responses in vivo.[41] ALW is a small molecule that can dissolve readily in H_2O or a standard buffer (PBS) and also be administered easily by vein. Moreover, the ALW peptide is likely to be physiologically stable; ALW lacks methionine, cysteine, and glutamine residues in its sequence, which are thought to be responsible for the oxidation, cyclization, and degradation of peptides, respectively.[84] Furthermore, ALW has a relatively neutral p*I* value (7.38), which can lead to less non-specific and unwanted interactions with other molecules.[41] Therefore, ALW peptide and its analogues are potential candidates in developing novel therapeutic approaches for treating SLE. In addition, our working assumption is that a combination of different peptides, selected by disparate approaches, may be necessary, since the pathogenic autoantibodies present in lupus are highly variable and cross-reactive.[41] Finally, in contrast to the models of peptide-induced autoimmunity described earlier where the peptide is given in an immunogenic setting (subcutaneously, in adjuvant), in a therapeutic context peptides given intravenously without adjuvant would not expected to be as immunogenic. Since peptides in the latter scenario are expected to have low toxicity, a combination approach might increase the efficacy of inhibition and improve clinical outcome.

Evidently, different peptides can be isolated by using anti-dsDNA antibodies of different origin as "bait." While there is not much similarity in structure between the peptides already identified, an interesting phenomenon is that tryptophan residue exists at similar positions in both DWEYSVWLSN (mouse antibody selected) and ALW (human antibody selected) peptides. The direct comparison of the relative blocking efficacy of these DNA-mimicking peptides would unfortunately not be revealing due to size differences. The fact that disparate peptides were isolated in different studies may be explained by the fact that different anti-dsDNA antibodies were used in the screening process. For example, DWEYSVWLSN and ASPVTARVLWKASHV were selected by a murine anti-dsDNA IgG2b monoclonal antibody and anti-dsDNA antibodies purified from human lupus sera, respectively.[80,87] Therefore, these anti-dsDNA antibodies might then display biased binding potential and potentially select different DNA-mimicking peptides. Moreover, the type and complexity of the specific phage library used may also affect the results in peptide screening.[41] Nevertheless, each of these peptides may bind to specific anti-DNA subsets, and it is possible that a better therapeutic response may be achieved by using several peptides in combination.

5.7 DEVELOPMENT OF NOVEL THERAPEUTIC APPROACHES TARGETING ANTI-dsDNA ANTIBODIES IN VIVO

Since the peptides bound by anti-dsDNA antibodies may block the binding of these pathogenic antibodies to self-antigens, the development of novel therapeutic approaches employing such peptides is attracting attention. Until now, several therapeutic peptides have been tested in murine models of SLE, with promising results in proof of concept studies.

DWEYS is a DNA-mimicking peptide selected by a pathogenic mouse monoclonal antibody (IgG2b, R4A clone). To assess whether the DWEYS peptide has potential for therapeutic application, 6- to 8-week-old SCID mice were injected intraperitoneally with purified R4A antibody and the DWEYS peptide, the latter of which was either in the L or D form.[80] Mice were sacrificed 16 h later, and kidney sections assessed for glomerular immunoglobulin deposition. Interestingly, the D form of DWEYS peptide significantly reduced R4A deposition in kidneys, whereas the L form of this peptide displayed little effect. Therefore, although it would also be important to ensure that the peptide did not stimulate an antidrug antibody response, a synthetic peptide DNA mimic did inhibit the deposition of anti-dsDNA antibodies in glomeruli in vivo.

Previous studies have showed that the DWEYS sequence can be found in both NR2A and NR2B subunits of the N-methyl-D-aspartate (NMDA) receptor in mouse and human.[85–87] Anti-dsDNA/DWEYS cross-reactive antibodies can be found in 40% of human lupus sera. Furthermore, this cross-reactive antibody fraction displays pathogenic potential for both brain and kidney.[88] Hence, neutralization of anti-dsDNA antibodies through a decoy peptide receptor may also prevent their pathogenic interaction with brain tissue antigens and attenuate neuropsychiatric lupus, which is believed at least in part to be antibody mediated. To enhance the therapeutic efficacy, the DWEYS peptide was modified to generate FISLE-412, a small peptidomimetic with improved affinity and selectivity.[88] FISLE-412 blocked DNA binding by monoclonal mouse (R4A) and human (G11) cross-reactive dsDNA/DWEYS antibodies by competitive ELISA. In addition, FISLE-412 abrogated tissue binding by either R4A or G11 to isolated kidney glomeruli. To test the inhibition of autoantibody-mediated neurotoxicity in vivo, C57BL/6 mice were injected into the hippocampus via a stereotaxic approach with either R4A or G11 that were preincubated with FILSE-412. Importantly, the FISLE-412-bound pathogenic antibodies failed to induce neurotoxic effects, as compared to the nonbound control antibodies. Moreover, the neuroprotective effect of FISLE-412 was greater than that afforded by the DWEYS peptide. The higher affinity of the engineered FISLE-412 for the pathogenic anti-dsDNA antibodies over the parent DWEYS peptide, in combination with enhanced structural stability and potentially oral availability, would make this reagent a promising novel approach for preventing the interaction of pathogenic anti-dsDNA/NMDAR antibodies with organs with affinity for these antibodies, namely, kidney and brain.

pCons is a 15-mer peptide (FIEWNKLRFRQGLEW) based on MHC class I and class II T cell determinants in the V_H region of a murine anti-dsDNA antibody,[89] which can block the binding of anti-DNA antibodies to self-antigens. Administration of pCons intravenously once a month to NZB×NZW F1 lupus mice, before disease was manifest, not only decreased the titers of lupus autoantibodies but also delayed the onset of nephritis and improved survival. A positive effect was also seen when treatment was initiated later on, treating older mice of this strain.[90] A striking effect observed was the ability of the peptide to induce tolerance in T cells and decrease the help provided by these cells for production of anti-dsDNA antibodies.[90] Finally, NZB×NZW F1 mice were vaccinated with B lymphocytes made transgenic for a gene coding a chimeric IgG1Fc-pCons construct,[91] with vaccinated mice exhibiting a delay in proteinuria and improvement in survival.

The studies reviewed here have therapeutic implications for other autoantibody-mediated diseases as well. In autoimmune conditions the autoantibody repertoire can be highly diverse and reactive with multiple antigens. Therefore, using peptides selected by a variety of techniques, perhaps in personalized combinations, may have improved efficacy in inhibiting the binding of autoantibodies to self-antigens, and subsequently a greater degree of clinical benefit.[41] A critical factor that may determine the efficacy of peptides administered orally, intravenously, or intraperitoneally is of course the in vivo half-life of the therapeutic and potential toxicity. Moreover, it will be important to ensure that these peptide therapeutics remain monomeric in circulation, possibly leading to lower immunogenicity and diminished immune complex formation with fewer unexpected side effects and toxicity.[92]

REFERENCES

1. Maroz N, Segal MS. Lupus nephritis and end-stage kidney disease. *Am J Med Sci* 2013;**346**:319–23.
2. Wang Z, Wang Y, Zhu R, Tian X, Xu D, Wang Q, Wu C, Zhang S, Zhao J, Zhao Y, Li M, Zeng X. Long-term survival and death causes of systemic lupus erythematosus in China: a systemic review of observational studies. *Medicine (Baltimore)* 2015;**94**:e794.
3. Wadee S, Tikly M, Hopley M. Causes and predictors of death in South Africans with systemic lupus erythematosus. *Rheumatology (Oxford)* 2007;**46**:1487–91.
4. Souza DC, Santo AH, Sato EI. Mortality profile related to systemic lupus erythematosus: a multiple cause-of-death analysis. *J Rheumatol* 2012;**39**:496–503.
5. Bernatsky S, Boivin JF, Joseph L, Manzi S, Ginzler E, Gladman DD, Urowitz M, Fortin PR, Petri M, Barr S, Gordon C, Bae SC, Isenberg D, Zoma A, Aranow C, Dooley MA, Nived O, Sturfelt G, Steinsson K, Alarcón G, Senécal JL, Zummer M, Hanly J, Ensworth S, Pope J, Edworthy S, Rahman A, Sibley J, El-Gabalawy H, McCarthy T, St Pierre Y, Clarke A, Ramsey-Goldman R. Mortality in systemic lupus erythematosus. *Arthritis Rheum* 2006;**54**:2550–7.
6. Yaniv G, Twig G, Shor DB, Furer A, Sherer Y, Mozes O, Komisar O, Slonimsky E, Klang E, Lotan E, Welt M, Marai I, Shina A, Amital H, Shoenfeld Y. A volcanic explosion of autoantibodies in systemic lupus erythematosus: a diversity of 180 different antibodies found in SLE patients. *Autoimmun Rev* 2015;**14**:75–9.
7. Perry D, Sang A, Yin Y, Zheng YY, Morel L. Murine models of systemic lupus erythematosus. *J Biomed Biotechnol* 2011;**2011**:271694.
8. Fu SM, Dai C, Zhao Z, Gaskin F. Anti-dsDNA antibodies are one of the many autoantibodies in systemic lupus erythematosus. *F1000Res* 2015;**4**(F1000 Faculty Rev):939.
9. Rekvig OP. Anti-dsDNA antibodies as a classification criterion and a diagnostic marker for systemic lupus erythematosus: critical remarks. *Clin Exp Immunol* 2015;**179**:5–10.
10. Xie C, Liang Z, Chang S, Mohan C. Use of a novel elution regimen reveals the dominance of polyreactive antinuclear autoantibodies in lupus kidneys. *Arthritis Rheum* 2003;**48**:2343–52.
11. Vlahakos DV, Foster MH, Adams S, Katz M, Ucci AA, Barrett KJ, Datta SK, Madaio MP. Anti-dsDNA antibodies form immune deposits at distinct glomerular and vascular sites. *Kidney Int* 1992;**41**:1690–700.
12. Foster MH, Fitzsimons MM. Lupus-like nephrotropic autoantibodies in non-autoimmune mice harboring an anti-basement membrane/anti-dsDNA Ig heavy chain transgene. *Mol Immunol* 1998;**35**:83–94.
13. Pan N, Amigues I, Lyman S, Duculan R, Aziz F, Crow MK, Kirou KA. A surge in anti-dsDNA titer predicts a severe lupus flare within six months. *Lupus* 2014;**23**:293–8.
14. Cardiel MH, Almagro RM. Steroid therapy in clinically stable but serologically active systemic lupus erythematosus prevents severe disease flares. *Expert Rev Clin Immunol* 2007;**3**:267–9.
15. Linnik MD, Hu JZ, Heilbrunn KR, Strand V, Hurley FL, Joh T. LJP 394 investigator consortium. Relationship between anti-double-stranded DNA antibodies and exacerbation of renal disease in patients with systemic lupus erythematosus. *Arthritis Rheum* 2005;**52**:1129–37.
16. Sherer Y, Gorstein A, Fritzler MJ, Shoenfeld Y. Autoantibody explosion in systemic lupus erythematosus: more than 100 different antibodies found in SLE patients. *Semin Arthritis Rheum* 2004;**34**:501–37.

17. Budhai L, Oh K, Davidson A. An in vitro assay for detection of glomerular binding IgG auto-antibodies in patients with systemic lupus erythematosus. *J Clin Invest* 1996;**98**:1585–93.
18. Zhao Z, Weinstein E, Tuzova M, Davidson A, Mundel P, Marambio P, Putterman C. Cross-reactivity of human lupus anti-dsDNA antibodies with alpha-actinin and nephritogenic potential. *Arthritis Rheum* 2005;**52**:522–30.
19. Yung S, Cheung KF, Zhang Q, Chan TM. Anti-dsDNA antibodies bind to mesangial annexin II in lupus nephritis. *J Am Soc Nephrol* 2010;**21**:1912–27.
20. Xia Y, Pawar RD, Nakouzi AS, Herlitz L, Broder A, Liu K, Goilav B, Fan M, Wang L, Li QZ, Casadevall A, Putterman C. The constant region contributes to the antigenic specificity and renal pathogenicity of murine anti-dsDNA antibodies. *J Autoimmun* 2012;**39**:398–411.
21. Yung S, Chan TM. Mechanisms of kidney injury in lupus nephritis—the role of anti-dsDNA antibodies. *Front Immunol* 2015;**6**:475.
22. Jang EJ, Nahm DH, Jang YJ. Mouse monoclonal autoantibodies penetrate mouse macro-phage cells and stimulate NF-kappaB activation and TNF-alpha release. *Immunol Lett* 2009;**124**:70–6.
23. Im SR, Im SW, Chung HY, Pravinsagar P, Jang YJ. Cell- and nuclear-penetrating anti-dsDNA autoantibodies have multiple arginines in CDR3 of VH and increase cellular level of pERK and Bcl-2 in mesangial cells. *Mol Immunol* 2015;**67**(2 Pt B):377–87.
24. Qing X, Pitashny M, Thomas DB, Barrat FJ, Hogarth MP, Putterman C. Pathogenic anti-dsDNA antibodies modulate gene expression in mesangial cells: involvement of HMGB1 in anti-dsDNA antibody-induced renal injury. *Immunol Lett* 2008;**121**:61–73.
25. Zhang Y, Yang J, Jiang S, Fang C, Xiong L, Cheng H, Xia Y. The lupus-derived anti-double-stranded DNA IgG contributes to myofibroblast-like phenotype in mesangial cells. *J Clin Immunol* 2012;**32**:1270–8.
26. Yung S, Tsang RC, Sun Y, Leung JK, Chan TM. Effect of human anti-dsDNA antibodies on proximal renal tubular epithelial cell cytokine expression: implications on tubulointerstitial inflammation in lupus nephritis. *J Am Soc Nephrol* 2005;**16**:3281–94.
27. Pisetsky DS. Standardization of anti-DNA antibody assays. *Immunol Res* 2013;**56**:420–4.
28. Stollar BD, Zon G, Pastor RW. A recognition site on synthetic helical oligonucleotides for monoclonal anti-native DNA autoantibody. *Proc Natl Acad Sci U S A* 1986;**83**:4469–73.
29. Alam K, Ali R. Human anti-DNA autoantibodies and induced antibodies against ROS-modified-DNA show similar antigenic binding characteristics. *Biochem Mol Biol Int* 1999;**47**:881–90.
30. Stollar BD. Molecular analysis of anti-DNA antibodies. *FASEB J* 1994;**8**:337–42.
31. Xia Y, Eryilmaz E, Zhang Q, Cowburn D, Putterman C. Anti-DNA antibody mediated catalysis is isotype dependent. *Mol Immunol* 2016;**69**:33–43.
32. Akberova NI, Zhmurov AA, Nevzorova TA, Litvinov RI. An anti-DNA antibody prefers damaged dsDNA over native. *J Biomol Struct Dyn* 2017;**35**(1):219–232. https://doi.org/10.1080/07391102.2015.1128979.
33. Tsuzaka K, Winkler TH, Kalden JR, Reichlin M. Autoantibodies to double-stranded (ds)DNA immunoprecipitate 18S ribosomal RNA by virtue of their interaction with ribosomal protein S1 and suppress in vitro protein synthesis. *Clin Exp Immunol* 1996;**106**:504–8.
34. Krasnorutskii MA, Buneva VN, Nevinsky GA. Antibodies against RNA hydrolyze RNA and DNA. *J Mol Recognit* 2008;**21**:338–47.
35. Servais G, Karmali R, Guillaume MP, Badot V, Duchateau J, Corazza F. Anti DNA antibodies are not restricted to a specific pattern of fluorescence on HEp2 cells. *Clin Chem Lab Med* 2009;**47**:543–9.
36. Franchin G, Son M, Kim SJ, Ben-Zvi I, Zhang J, Diamond B. Anti-DNA antibodies cross-react with C1q. *J Autoimmun* 2013;**44**:34–9.

37. Zou X, Cheng H, Zhang Y, Fang C, Xia Y. The antigen-binding fragment of anti-double-stranded DNA IgG enhances F-actin formation in mesangial cells by binding to alpha-actinin-4. *Exp Biol Med (Maywood)* 2012;**237**:1023–31.

38. Yoshioka H, Yoshida H, Usui T, Sung M, Ko K, Takeuchi E, Kita T, Sugiyama T. Spontaneous development of anti-collagen type II antibodies with NTA, and anti-DNA antibodies in senescence-accelerated mice. *Autoimmunity* 1993;**14**:215–20.

39. Lake RA, Morgan A, Henderson B, Staines NA. A key role for fibronectin in the sequential binding of native dsDNA and monoclonal anti-DNA antibodies to components of the extracellular matrix: its possible significance in glomerulonephritis. *Immunology* 1985;**54**:389–95.

40. Spellerberg MB, Chapman CJ, Mockridge CI, Isenberg DA, Stevenson FK. Dual recognition of lipid A and DNA by human antibodies encoded by the VH4-21 gene: a possible link between infection and lupus. *Hum Antibodies Hybridomas* 1995;**6**:52–6.

41. Xia Y, Eryilmaz E, Der E, Pawar RD, Guo X, Cowburn D, Putterman C. A peptide mimic blocks the cross reaction of anti-DNA antibodies with glomerular antigens. *Clin Exp Immunol* 2016;**183**:369–79.

42. Beger E, Deocharan B, Edelman M, Erblich B, Gu Y, Putterman C. A peptide DNA surrogate accelerates autoimmune manifestations and nephritis in lupus-prone mice. *J Immunol* 2002;**168**:3617–26.

43. Zhang W, Reichlin M. A peptide DNA surrogate that binds and inhibits anti-dsDNA antibodies. *Clin Immunol* 2005;**117**:214–20.

44. Sun Y, Fong KY, Chung MC, Yao ZJ. Peptide mimicking antigenic and immunogenic epitope of double-stranded DNA in systemic lupus erythematosus. *Int Immunol* 2001;**13**:223–32.

45. Sibille P, Ternynck T, Nato F, Buttin G, Strosberg D, Avrameas A. Mimotopes of polyreactive anti-DNA antibodies identified using phage-display peptide libraries. *Eur J Immunol* 1997;**27**:1221–8.

46. Dieker JW, Sun YJ, Jacobs CW, Putterman C, Monestier M, Muller S, van der Vlag J, Berden JH. Mimotopes for lupus-derived anti-DNA and nucleosome-specific autoantibodies selected from random peptide phage display libraries: facts and follies. *J Immunol Methods* 2005;**296**:83–93.

47. Torres M, Casadevall A. The immunoglobulin constant region contributes to affinity and specificity. *Trends Immunol* 2008;**29**:91–7.

48. Janda A, Bowen A, Greenspan NS, Casadevall A. Ig constant region effects on variable region structure and function. *Front Microbiol* 2016;**7**:22.

49. Janda A, Eryilmaz E, Nakouzi A, Pohl MA, Bowen A, Casadevall A. Variable region identical IgA and IgE to Cryptococcus neoformans capsular polysaccharide manifest specificity differences. *J Biol Chem* 2015;**290**:12090–100.

50. Bijl M, Dijstelbloem HM, Oost WW, Bootsma H, Derksen RH, Aten J, Limburg PC, Kallenberg CG. IgG subclass distribution of autoantibodies differs between renal and extra-renal relapses in patients with systemic lupus erythematosus. *Rheumatology (Oxford)* 2002;**41**:62–7.

51. Ebling F, Hahn BH. Restricted subpopulations of DNA antibodies in kidneys of mice with systemic lupus. Comparison of antibodies in serum and renal eluates. *Arthritis Rheum* 1980;**23**:392–403.

52. Baudino L, Azeredo da Silveira S, Nakata M, Izui S. Molecular and cellular basis for pathogenicity of autoantibodies: lessons from murine monoclonal autoantibodies. *Springer Semin Immunopathol* 2006;**28**:175–84.

53. Xia Y, Janda A, Eryilmaz E, Casadevall A, Putterman C. The constant region affects antigen binding of antibodies to DNA by altering secondary structure. *Mol Immunol* 2013;**56**:28–37.

54. Cooper LJ, Shikhman AR, Glass DD, Kangisser D, Cunningham MW, Greenspan NS. Role of heavy chain constant domains in antibody-antigen interaction. Apparent specificity differences among streptococcal IgG antibodies expressing identical variable domains. *J Immunol* 1993;**150**:2231–42.

55. Pritsch O, Magnac C, Dumas G, Bouvet JP, Alzari P, Dighiero G. Can isotype switch modulate antigen-binding affinity and influence clonal selection? *Eur J Immunol* 2000;**30**:3387–95.

56. Tudor D, Yu H, Maupetit J, Drillet AS, Bouceba T, Schwartz-Cornil I, et al. Isotype modulates epitope specificity, affinity, and antiviral activities of anti-HIV-1 human broadly neutralizing 2F5 antibody. *Proc Natl Acad Sci U S A* 2012;**109**:12680–5.

57. Janda A, Casadevall A. Circular dichroism reveals evidence of coupling between immunoglobulin constant and variable region secondary structure. *Mol Immunol* 2010;**47**:1421–5.

58. Janda A, Eryilmaz E, Nakouzi A, Cowburn D, Casadevall A. Variable region identical immunoglobulins differing in isotype express different paratopes. *J Biol Chem* 2012;**287**:35409–17.

59. Victora GD, Nussenzweig MC. Germinal centers. *Annu Rev Immunol* 2012;**30**:429–57.

60. O'Keefe TL, Datta SK, Imanishi-Kari T. Cationic residues in pathogenic anti-DNA autoantibodies arise by mutations of a germ-line gene that belongs to a large VH gene subfamily. *Eur J Immunol* 1992;**22**:619–24.

61. Tanner JJ, Komissarov AA, Deutscher SL. Crystal structure of an antigen-binding fragment bound to single-stranded DNA. *J Mol Biol* 2001;**314**:807–22.

62. Stanfield RL, Eilat D. Crystal structure determination of anti-DNA Fab A52. *Proteins* 2014;**82**(1678):1674.

63. Li Z, Schettino EW, Padlan EA, Ikematsu H, Casali P. Structure-function analysis of a lupus anti-DNA autoantibody: central role of the heavy chain complementarity-determining region 3 Arg in binding of double- and single-stranded DNA. *Eur J Immunol* 2000;**30**:2015–26.

64. Aas-Hanssen K, Funderud A, Thompson KM, B3 B, Munthe LA. Idiotype-specific Th cells support oligoclonal expansion of anti-dsDNA B cells in mice with lupus. *J Immunol* 2014;**193**:2691–8.

65. Jang YJ, Stollar BD. Anti-DNA antibodies: aspects of structure and pathogenicity. *Cell Mol Life Sci* 2003;**60**:309–20.

66. Kieber-Emmons T, Foster MH, Williams WV, Madaio MP. Structural properties of a subset of nephritogenic anti-DNA antibodies. *Immunol Res* 1994;**13**:172–85.

67. Putterman C, Limpanasithikul W, Edelman M, Diamond B. The double edged sword of the immune response: mutational analysis of a murine anti-pneumococcal, anti-DNA antibody. *J Clin Invest* 1996;**97**:2251–9.

68. Ou Z, Bottoms CA, Henzl MT, Tanner JJ. Impact of DNA hairpin folding energetics on antibody-ssDNA association. *J Mol Biol* 2007;**374**:1029–40.

69. Paul S, Planque SA, Nishiyama Y, Hanson CV, Massey RJ. Nature nurture of catalytic antibodies. *Adv Exp Med Biol* 2012;**750**:56–75.

70. Gololobov GV, Rumbley CA, Rumbley JN, Schourov DV, Makarevich OI, Gabibov AG, Voss Jr. EW, Rodkey LS. DNA hydrolysis by monoclonal anti-ssDNA autoantibody BV 04-01: origins of catalytic activity. *Mol Immunol* 1997;**34**:1083–93.

71. Ponomarenko NA, Durova OM, Vorobiev II, Aleksandrova ES, Telegin GB, Chamborant OG, Sidorik LL, Suchkov SV, Alekberova ZS, Gnuchev NV, Gabibov AG. Catalytic antibodies in clinical and experimental pathology: human and mouse models. *J Immunol Methods* 2002;**269**:197–211.

72. Nevinsky GA, Buneva VN. Natural catalytic antibodies in norm, autoimmune, viral, and bacterial diseases. *Sci World J* 2010;**10**:1203–33.

73. Rao DN, Wootla B. Catalytic antibodies: concept and promise. *Resonance* 2007;**12**:6–21.

74. Shuster AM, Gololobov GV, Kvashuk OA, Bogomolova AE, Smirnov IV, Gabibov AG. DNA hydrolyzing autoantibodies. *Science* 1992;**256**:665–7.

75. Nevinsky GA, Buneva VN. Human catalytic RNA- and DNA-hydrolyzing antibodies. *J Immunol Methods* 2002;**269**:235–49.

76. Kostrikina IA, Kolesova ME, Orlovskaya IA, Buneva VN, Nevinsky GA. Diversity of DNA-hydrolyzing antibodies from the sera of autoimmune-prone MRL/MpJ-lpr mice. *J Mol Recognit* 2011;**24**:557–69.

77. Kostrikina IA, Odintsova ES, Buneva VN, Nevinsky GA. Systemic lupus erythematosus: molecular cloning and analysis of recombinant DNase monoclonal κ light chain NGK-1. *Int Immunol* 2014;**26**:439–50.

78. Kozyr AV, Sashchenko LP, Kolesnikov AV, Zelenova NA, Khaidukov SV, Ignatova AN, Bobik TV, Gabibov AG, Alekberova ZS, Suchkov SV, Gnuchev NV. Anti-DNA autoantibodies reveal toxicity to tumor cell lines. *Immunol Lett* 2002;**80**:41–7.

79. Mouratou B, Rouyre S, Guesdon JL. A method for the detection and screening of catalytic anti-DNA antibodies. *J Immunol Methods* 2002;**269**:147–55.

80. Gaynor B, Putterman C, Valadon P, Spatz L, Scharff MD, Diamond B. Peptide inhibition of glomerular deposition of an anti-DNA antibody. *Proc Natl Acad Sci U S A* 1997;**94**:1955–60.

81. Putterman C, Deocharan B, Diamond B. Molecular analysis of the autoantibody response in peptide-induced autoimmunity. *J Immunol* 2000;**164**:2542–9.

82. Putterman C, Diamond B. Immunization with a peptide surrogate for double-stranded DNA (dsDNA) induces autoantibody production and renal immunoglobulin deposition. *J Exp Med* 1998;**188**:29–38.

83. Deocharan B, Qing X, Beger E, Putterman C. Antigenic triggers and molecular targets for anti-double-stranded DNA antibodies. *Lupus* 2002;**11**:865–71.

84. Hoeppe S, Schreiber TD, Planatscher H, Zell A, Templin MF, Stoll D, Joos TO, Poetz O. Targeting peptide termini, a novel immunoaffinity approach to reduce complexity in mass spectrometric protein identification. *Mol Cell Proteomics* 2011;**10**:M110.002857.

85. Katz JB, Limpanasithikul W, Diamond B. Mutational analysis of an autoantibody: differential binding and pathogenicity. *J Exp Med* 1994;**180**:925–32.

86. Shefner R, Kleiner G, Turken A, Papazian L, Diamond B. A novel class of anti-DNA antibodies identified in BALB/c mice. *J Exp Med* 1991;**173**:287–96.

87. DeGiorgio LA, Konstantinov KN, Lee SC, Hardin JA, Volpe BT, Diamond B. A subset of lupus anti-DNA antibodies cross-reacts with the NR2 glutamate receptor in systemic lupus erythematosus. *Nat Med* 2001;**7**:1189–93.

88. Bloom O, Cheng KF, He M, Papatheodorou A, Volpe BT, Diamond B, Al-Abed Y. Generation of a unique small molecule peptidomimetic that neutralizes lupus autoantibody activity. *Proc Natl Acad Sci U S A* 2011;**108**:10255–9.

89. Sthoeger Z, Sharabi A, Mozes E. Novel approaches to the development of targeted therapeutic agents for systemic lupus erythematosus. *J Autoimmun* 2014;**54**:60–71.

90. Hahn BH, Singh RR, Wong WK, Tsao BP, Bulpitt K, Ebling FM. Treatment with a consensus peptide based on amino acid sequences in autoantibodies prevents T cell activation by autoantigens and delays disease onset in murine lupus. *Arthritis Rheum* 2001;**44**:432–41.

91. Ferrera F, Fenoglio D, Cutolo M, Balbi G, Parodi A, Battaglia F, Kalli F, Barone D, Indiveri F, Criscuolo D, Filaci G. Early and repeated IgG1Fc-pCons chimera vaccinations (GX101) improve the outcome in SLE-prone mice. *Clin Exp Med* 2015;**15**:255–60.

92. Diamond B, Bloom O, Al Abed Y, Kowal C, Huerta PT, Volpe BT. Moving towards a cure: blocking pathogenic antibodies in systemic lupus erythematosus. *J Intern Med* 2011;**269**:36–44.

Chapter 6

The Role of the Constant Region in Antibody-Antigen Interactions: Redefining the Modular Model of Immunoglobulin Structure

Anthony Bowen*, Arturo Casadevall†

*Albert Einstein College of Medicine, New York, NY, United States, †Johns Hopkins Bloomberg School of Public Health, Baltimore, MD, United States

6.1 INTRODUCTION

In 1890, Emil von Behring and Shibasaburo Kitasato discovered that a substance in the serum of immunized animals was protective against diphtheria and tetanus toxins, later leading to use of immune sera as the first passive immunotherapies and, for von Behring, the first Nobel Prize in Physiology or Medicine in 1901.[1] The activity of their antitoxin was traced to the gamma globulins, named for their position following serum electrophoresis, and eventually to antibody or immunoglobulin molecules in 1939.[2] Immunoglobulins are glycoproteins produced by B lymphocytes in all vertebrates as an essential part of the immune response. In more than 120 years following the discovery of antitoxin, enormous progress has been made in describing antibody structure and understanding the complex mechanisms of antibody production and function. In general, immunoglobulins function by recognizing and binding foreign molecules, both neutralizing them independently and enabling recognition by other immune components. Immunological canon divides antibody molecules into two functionally independent segments: (1) a variable region that binds foreign molecules, or antigens, and (2) a constant region that is recognized by downstream components of the immune response, which proceed to carry out a variety of effector functions. In this chapter, we will discuss the large and growing body of work showing that antibody constant and variable regions are not, in fact, functionally independent. The idea that conformational changes in the constant

Structural Biology in Immunology. https://doi.org/10.1016/B978-0-12-803369-2.00006-1

region can affect specificity of an antibody for its cognate antigen is not a new one. Here, we trace the roots of this idea in the scientific literature and discuss the converse, the notion that antigen binding can cause conformational changes in the constant region. Through an analysis of the available evidence, we will highlight the effects of the constant region on antibody-antigen interactions and argue that the classic view of antibody regions as functionally independent units fails to fully reflect the complex and important roles these fascinating molecules play in the immune system.

6.2 IMMUNOGLOBULIN STRUCTURE

Reviewing the structural composition of the immunoglobulin molecule is a useful prerequisite before discussing their diverse functions. The basic antibody template is a Y-shaped unit consisting of two identical polypeptide heavy (H) chains and two identical polypeptide light (L) chains joined together through disulfide bonds (Fig. 6.1). A complete immunoglobulin is produced as either monomers or oligomers of this Y-shaped template. The H and L chains have a modular construction made up of discrete protein domains. The L chain contains two discrete domains, while the H chain contains four to five domains. Each H and L chain contains a constant (C_H or C_L) and variable (V_H or V_L) region. Antibody V regions consist of the first protein domain at the amino-terminus of each polypeptide chain and are responsible for binding cognate antigens, while C regions include the remaining domains and engage host cellular and molecular components of the immune system.

In mammals, antibodies exist in five major classes or isotypes possessing distinct structures and functions (Table 6.1). The five main antibody isotypes (IgG, IgM, IgA, IgE, and IgD) are determined by five different C_H types (gamma γ, mu μ, alpha α, epsilon ε, and delta δ, respectively). The various C_H classes differ in size and structure, with γ, α, and δ consisting of three discrete domains (C_{H1-3}), and μ and ε consisting of four discrete domains (C_{H1-4}). In the γ, α, and δ classes, the C_{H1} and C_{H2} domains are separated by a flexible polypeptide hinge region, which forms disulfide bonds with the hinge region of the neighboring H chain. The number of disulfide bonds and the length of the hinge vary by isotype. The μ and ε classes lack a hinge region, making IgM and IgE antibodies less flexible than other isotypes. Some C_H variants have a number of distinct subclasses in different mammalian species. We will focus on human and mouse antibodies as these are the most widely studied and utilized. Humans produce two IgA subclasses (IgA1 and IgA2) and four IgG subclasses (IgG1, IgG2, IgG3, and IgG4). Mice produce only one type of IgA and five subclasses of IgG (IgG1, IgG2a, IgG2b, IgG2c, and IgG3). Antibodies also exist with two different L chain types, known as kappa (κ) and lambda (λ), that do not alter the isotype. Several λ C_L subtypes are found in both humans and mice; however, most serum antibodies contain the κ C_L. The C_L region consists of a single protein domain and typically contains a disulfide linkage to the C_{H1}

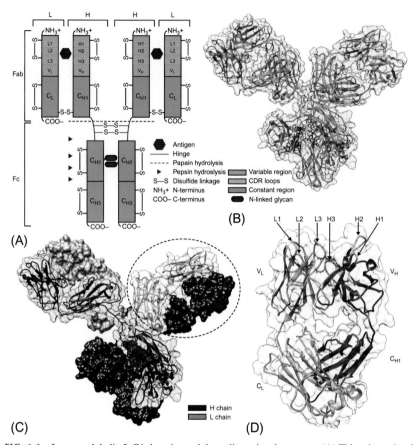

FIG. 6.1   Immunoglobulin IgG1 domains and three-dimensional structure. (A) This schematic of an IgG1 illustrates the molecule's H and L chains, discrete protein domains, disulfide linkages, and CDR regions. Papain hydrolysis produces two Fab fragments and one Fc fragment, while pepsin hydrolysis produces one F(ab')$_2$ fragment and several fragments of the Fc. Glycosylation is shown at asparagine 297. (B) The X-ray crystal structure of an intact IgG1 is shown and colored by C and V region with the CDR loops highlighted (PDBID: 1IGY).[3] Disulfide linkages are shown as sticks and colored *yellow*, while glycans are colored *purple*. The β strands and sheets of the immunoglobulin fold are visible in the ribbon structure. (C) This view of the same antibody shows the H chains colored *red* and L chains colored *gray*. The dashed circle indicates one of the Fabs, which is shown in panel D. (D) A side view of one of the IgG1 Fabs with the H chain colored *red* and the L chain colored *gray*. Surfaces of the C$_L$ and C$_{H1}$ domains are colored *blue*, while the V$_H$ and V$_L$ surfaces are *green*. CDR loops are labeled 1–3 for the L and H chains and colored *gold*.

domain of the H chain. Antibodies of each isotype are produced as both serum proteins and as monomeric membrane-bound molecules that form part of the B cell receptor. Monomeric IgG comprises the vast majority of antibody found in the serum (Table 6.1).[4–6] Serum IgM is produced as either a pentamer linked by an additional peptide joining (J) chain, or as a hexamer, leading this isotype to have a very high avidity for antigen. While IgA found in the serum is typically

TABLE 6.1 Human Antibody Isotypes and Their Subtypes Have Numerous Structural and Functional Differences[4,5].

Isotype Subtype	Oligomerization	Abundance	[Serum] (mg/mL)	Molecular Weight (kDa)	Half-life (days)	Carbohydrates	Functions
IgG	Monomers	75%	10		23	3%	Secondary response
IgG1		67% IgG		150			
IgG2		22% IgG		150			
IgG3		7% IgG		170	8		
IgG4		4% IgG		150			
IgM	Pentamers (+ J chain); Hexamers	10%	1.2	950 (pentamer)	5	12%	Primary response
IgA	Monomers (serum); Dimers, rarely trimers, tetramers for sIgA (+ SC, + J chain)	15%	2	160 (monomer)	5–6	7.5%	Mucosal response
IgA1		90% serum IgA					
IgA2		10% serum IgA					
IgD	Monomers	<0.5%	0.04	180	2.8	12%	Homeostasis
IgE	Monomers	<0.01%	3.00E−04	190	2.5	12%	Allergy

monomeric and makes up about 15% of the total antibody content, more of this isotype is produced than all of the others combined and secreted across mucosal membranes and in bodily secretions as secretory IgA (sIgA). Usually, sIgA is produced as a dimer with its monomers attached via the J chain. It is also typically linked to another peptide called the secretory component (SC). However, sIgA can also rarely be found as monomers, trimers, or tetramers. IgE and IgD are normally found in the serum at very low levels as monomers.

All immunoglobulin V and C region protein domains share a similar structure. Each domain contains approximately 110–130 amino acids with a molecular mass of 12–13 kDa and consists of two β sheets packed against each other into a β sandwich with a hydrophobic core. The two β sheets are connected by a single disulfide bond and are made up of antiparallel β strands joined by loops. This characteristic domain is known as the immunoglobulin fold and is present in many other key proteins of the immune system, which together constitute the immunoglobulin superfamily (IgSF) of proteins. V region immunoglobulin domains are slightly larger than those of the C region, containing an extra loop and two additional β strands for a total of nine. Three loops in each V region domain contain hypervariable amino acid sequences known as complementarity-determining regions (CDRs), which form a binding surface. The remarkably plastic paratope, or combining site, of an antibody is generated by the combination of all six CDRs from the V_H and V_L domains when the H and L chains are joined. Amino acids in the V domain that do not form part of a CDR are categorized as framework (FR) residues.

Functional fragments and mimics of antibodies are extensively studied in the literature as a means of dissecting the roles played by immunoglobulins, as possible therapeutic agents, and as molecular research tools. Limited digestion of immunoglobulin molecules with papain, a cysteine protease found in the papaya fruit, hydrolyzes the immunoglobulin hinge region between the C_{H1} domain and the disulfide bonds that join the H chains. This digestion yields two identical Fab fragments (fragment antigen binding) and one Fc fragment (fragment crystallizable, named as such because it was found to readily crystalize). An Fab has a molecular mass of approximately 50 kDa and contains the V_H, V_L, C_{H1}, and C_L domains. The orientation of the Fab's two V domains relative to its two C domains is referred to as the elbow angle and is known to vary widely. The Fc consists of two joined H chains missing the V_H and C_{H1} domains. The terms Fab and Fc are frequently used to refer to the respective regions of intact immunoglobulin molecules in addition to the fragments generated by papain digestion. Limited antibody digestion with pepsin typically hydrolyzes immunoglobulins below the disulfide bonds in the hinge region and at several locations throughout the C_{H2} domain. This leads to the generation of one 100 kDa F(ab')$_2$ fragment consisting of two Fabs joined by the disulfide bonds in the hinge. The largest remaining piece of the Fc region is referred to as the pFc' fragment.

Immunoglobulins, like many other serum proteins, are normally glycosylated by the covalent attachment of sugar residues to certain amino acids. The amount, structure, and sites of attachment of carbohydrate chains, or glycans, to immunoglobulins vary widely by species and isotype. Even immunoglobulins with identical protein sequences produced by the same B cell can differ in their glycan modifications, yielding distinct glycoforms of the same antibody. Glycan chains attached to antibodies usually consist of D-galactose (Gal), N-acetyl-D-galactosamine (GalNAc), N-acetyl-D-glucosamine (GlcNAc), L-fucose (Fuc), D-mannose (Man), and N-acetylneuraminic acid (NeuAc) sugar residues.[4] Most commonly, oligosaccharide chains are attached to immunoglobulins at asparagine residues as N-linked glycans, but they can also be linked to the hydroxyl groups of serine or threonine residues as O-linked glycans. Most antibody glycosylation occurs in the heavy chain constant region and can be asymmetric across an immunoglobulin's two H chains, leading to an even greater increase in antibody structural diversity. The major site of carbohydrate attachment in IgGs is at asparagine 297 in the C_{H2} domain; however, other glycan modifications are occasionally found at a number of different positions in the V and C regions of the H and L chains.[7] Glycosylation of IgG at asparagine 297 is necessary for complement activation and interaction of the immunoglobulin with cellular Fc receptors.[8,9] Murine IgG3 has a second glycosylation site at asparagine 471 in the C_{H3} domain. The glycans attached at this position have been shown to be important for the ability of IgG3 molecules to self-associate.[4,10] Furthermore, glycosylation of the V region has also been shown to affect the affinity of antibodies for antigen by altering the conformations of amino acids in the paratope.[11]

The modular nature of the immunoglobulin molecule along with advances in molecular biology has facilitated the generation of a wide variety of recombinant antibody mimics and derivatives.[12] One of the most commonly studied of these is the single-chain Fv (scFv), which consists of the V_H and V_L domains joined by a synthetic peptide linker. Another immunoglobulin derivative with widespread potential use is the bispecific antibody, which is generated by combining different H and L chains to create two distinct binding surfaces on each antibody monomer. Some species produce antibody variants that lack the L chain entirely. In camelids, a large proportion of produced antibodies are so-called heavy-chain immunoglobulins (hcIgs) that arise through deletion of the C_{H1} domain and modification of the V_H domain, thus preventing L chain association.[13] Cartilaginous fish, on the other hand, produce a heavy-chain antibody known as the immunoglobulin new- antigen receptor (IgNAR) with significant structural differences in the V_H and C_H regions compared to those of mammals.[14] The generation of single-domain antibodies (sdAbs), which consist of only the V_H domain, was initially made possible by the discovery of IgNAR and hcIg molecules. More recently, sdAbs have been generated from the V_H domains and, less commonly, the V_L domains of other species.[15,16]

The major function of immunoglobulin molecules is to specifically recognize and bind to cognate antigens. Because the antibody paratope emerges from the combined CDR loops of both the H and L chains, each Y-shaped monomer contains two identical binding sites at the ends of its two Fabs (Fig. 6.1). The physical interaction of an antigen and a single antibody combining site begins with the diffusion-limited orientation of the two molecular surfaces and is subsequently driven by a variety of noncovalent forces including hydrogen bonding, electrostatic and hydrophobic interactions, aromatic pi stacking, and van der Waals forces. The relative contributions of these forces to the strength of the interaction are dependent on the antigen-antibody pair and can be heavily modified by changes to the amino acids present in the CDR loops. Intrinsic antibody affinity refers to the strength of the interaction between one antibody paratope and one antigen epitope. Intrinsic affinity can also be modified by a number of additional factors including temperature, pressure, pH, ionic strength, and antibody or antigen concentration. Functional affinity, or avidity, reflects the effective affinity of multiple joined antibody paratopes for a multivalent antigen. Since IgG, IgE, and IgD are primarily monomeric, their 2 paratopes lead to significantly lower functional affinities than the 4 paratopes of dimeric IgA or the 10 paratopes of pentameric IgM.

6.3 THE MODULAR ANTIBODY MODEL

The classic view of antibody structure-function relationships was born in the 1950s and 1960s, when new experimental techniques facilitated the purification and sequence determination of biological proteins, thus enabling the first detailed structural glimpses of immunoglobulins. The model was then reinforced and refined over the subsequent four decades with experiments made possible through ongoing technological innovations. Beginning in 1950, Rodney Porter was the first to show that the enzyme papain hydrolyzed IgG molecules into three fragments with distinct functions. Two of the fragments retained antigen-binding capability (Fabs) but were no longer able to precipitate antigen. The larger third fragment was readily crystallizable (Fc) but was unable to bind antigen.[17,18] At around the same time, Gerald Edelman, who together with Porter was awarded the 1972 Nobel Prize in Physiology or Medicine, succeeded in dissociating IgG into its constituent heavy and light chains by reducing the disulfide bonds that normally hold the polypeptide chains together.[19] Edelman recognized that the IgG fragments produced by disulfide reduction were orthogonal to those produced by Porter's enzymatic digestion and later succeeded in determining the complete covalent layout and amino acid sequence of an antibody molecule.[20] With the linear arrangement of the immunoglobulin molecule in hand, Edelman was able to draw conclusions in a 1969 paper about the structure-function relationships of antibodies that would soon become central tenets in immunology:

> *One of the most striking features of the immunoglobulin molecule that emerges from the completed sequence is the sharp demarcation of its polypeptide chains into linearly connected regions that are associated with different functions.*

Variation in the sequences of paired V_H and V_L regions for the function of antigen binding in the selective immune response, and at the same time, conservation of sequence in C_H and C_L regions for other immunological functions appear to require special genetic and evolutionary mechanisms. ...C regions, like enzymes, may have evolved to interact with specific molecules, e.g., those of the complement system.[20]

On the heels of Edelmen's prescient words, Elvin Kabat—who had earlier demonstrated that gamma globulins were antibodies—and others carried out pioneering work characterizing the diversity of light- and heavy-chain amino acid sequences. His studies were the first to identify hypervariable CDR regions in the V_H and V_L domains and to conclude that they were evolutionarily selected for binding diverse antigen.[21–23] From these studies, the modular model of antibody function was proposed as a demarcation of immunoglobulins into antigen-binding variable regions and conserved constant regions that confer immune effector functions. It is remarkable that so many details about antibody function could be inferred from the arrangement of the molecule's polypeptide chains and the activity of its hydrolyzed fragments. In the subsequent decades, the application of new tools would shed light on antibody production, diversity, structure, and function, further cementing the modular antibody model.

Following the determination of numerous antibody protein sequences, an extensive debate began surrounding the question of how highly variable V regions could be encoded in the germline and also linked to the conserved C region. Beginning in 1974, Susumu Tonegawa published a series of experiments showing that the genes encoding antibody V_L and C_L regions were separated in the embryonic genome, but close together in the genomes of somatic antibody-producing cells.[24–27] In these differentiated cells, recombination was postulated to be responsible for the joining of a single variable (V), joining (J), and constant (C) gene to create a complete light chain sequence. Tonegawa also concluded that in these differentiated cells, some mechanism of allelic exclusion must be operating to prevent multiple V regions from being expressed by the same cell. While Tonegawa's first experiments focused on light chain genes, it would only be a few years before the discovery of similar genetic mechanisms underlying the generation of heavy chains. Leroy Hood, Tonegawa, and others showed in a number of papers that V_H regions are generated by the somatic recombination of three heavy chain V, J, and diversity (D) genes.[28–30] The VDJ gene segment was shown to become linked to a heavy chain C gene that determined the antibody class and subtype. These observations opened the door for future determination of the mechanism of class-switch recombination, where a single VDJ gene segment is recombined with a new C gene to generate antibodies possessing the same antigen-binding domain but a different isotype.[30] The observed numbers of V, D, and J germline genes could not account for the full diversity of the antibody repertoire, leading Tonegawa and others to conclude that some somatic process, now known to be somatic hypermutation, operates on the V(D)J gene segments to further increase their sequence diversity. This series of pivotal discoveries earned Tonegawa the 1987 Nobel Prize in Physiology or Medicine and further cemented the modular concept of antibody molecules by describing distinct germline locations and genetic mechanisms for C and V regions to go along with the distinct immunological functions they were thought to provide.

Direct structural evidence for the isolation of V and C region functions came on heels of advances in X-ray crystallography. Early low-resolution studies of Fc fragments and intact immunoglobulins confirmed the existence of three globular regions—two Fabs and one Fc—connected by a flexible hinge.[31] The separation of relatively rigid Fab and Fc regions by the hinge was considered consistent with their apparent separation of functions. The hinge region was viewed as a physical and functional spacer between the workhorse domains of the immunoglobulin molecule. Subsequent high-resolution structures revealed the antiparallel beta sheets of the immunoglobulin fold and the colocalization of hypervariable loops, or CDRs, surrounding the Fab's antigen-binding site.[31,32] The modular view of antibody structure was reinforced two decades later in the late 1990s with the publication of high-resolution structures of intact immunoglobulins.[3,33] The spatial proximity of the hypervariable CDRs to one another and to bound haptens illustrated their role in forming the antibody-binding site for diverse antigen, proving Kabat's earlier hypothesis. A growing body of structural studies in the late 1980s and 1990s, using both X-ray diffraction and nuclear magnetic resonance (NMR), led to the characterization of the antibody-antigen interaction as an "induced fit," where the conformations of peptide backbones and side chains in the CDR loops were rearranged upon antigen binding.[34–41]

Following initial observations in 1959, it was known that antibody-antigen complexes were ingested even more readily than unbound antibody by phagocytic cells bearing Fc receptors.[42] This observation initially led many to hypothesize that intramolecular signaling was responsible, where conformational changes propagated to the Fc region following antigen binding causing an increased affinity for cellular Fc receptors.[43] Throughout the second half of the 20th century, a wealth of experimental techniques were used to probe structural changes in immunoglobulins upon binding antigen. Many of these studies yielded negative results that were consistent with the view that V and C regions functioned independently but could not explain the differing Fc receptor affinities for bound and unbound antibodies. Hapten studies of crystal structures and antibodies in solution showed no evidence of Fab or Fc conformational changes upon antigen binding.[33,44–48] Numerous circular dichroism studies of antibody-hapten complexes showed no changes in optical rotation of bound vs unbound antibodies.[49–52] While one of these studies did observe an effect with multivalent antigens, it was attributed to the complexation of antibody molecules rather than any conformational changes in the immunoglobulins themselves.[51] Low-resolution electron microscopy studies showed that the conformation of immunoglobulin domains remained constant following antigen binding; however, they also indicated that the two Fab regions of an IgG were flexible in relation to one another with internal angles ranging from 10 to 180 degrees.[53,54] This remarkable flexibility was generally attributed to the hinge region and was taken as an evidence against the idea that conformational changes in the Fab and Fc regions could influence one another. Later work by Oi et al. revealed that the flexibility of the hinge varied in immunoglobulins with the same V regions but varying isotypes, but found no differences in flexibility between bound and unbound antibodies of the same isotype.[55] Interestingly, this study also described a correlation between complement fixation and hinge flexibility, with one offered explanation being the transmission of conformational changes between the Fab and Fc regions. The concept of the hinge as a "loose tether" was more recently reinforced by the publication of the first intact human IgG crystal structure.[56] If the hypothesis of conformational changes following antigen binding was true, one manifestation could be an allosteric effect on the second antibody combining site following antigen interaction with the first. Several groups using rabbit and human antibodies compared binding affinities for whole antibody preparations and preparations of separated Fab and Fc fragments following papain digestion, finding no significant differences between the two.[57–59] In combination, these studies suggested that the interaction of hapten with one combining site had no effect on the conformation or affinity of the other site. The preponderance of negative data in conformational studies of bound vs unbound antibodies ultimately led to increasing doubts about the possibility for intramolecular signaling in the immunoglobulin.

6.4 EVIDENCE FOR INTRAMOLECULAR SIGNALING UPON ANTIGEN BINDING

Not all of the early research on conformational changes in bound antibodies produced negative results. In the 1970s, one study showed significant differences in the circular dichroic spectra of several rabbit antibodies following hapten binding, suggesting conformational changes in the antibodies.[60] Another group showed a slight increase in the sedimentation coefficient of a rabbit IgG following interaction of the antibody with a hapten.[61] This result indicated that the antibody adopted a more compact structure following hapten binding, which contrasted with prior electron microscopy data showing the separation of Fab regions upon interaction with a larger multivalent antigen.[53] Another set of experiments carried out by Ashman, Kaplan, and Metzger attempted to identify whether any conformational changes occur in human IgM following hapten binding.[62] Their work showed no changes in the circular dichroic spectra of human IgM bound to haptens. However, hydrogen-exchange experiments with tritiated water showed the presence of trapped hydrogen atoms in the immunoglobulin following antigen binding. This was taken to indicate either a conformational change or a steric blocking of antibody residues by the hapten. Ashman and Metzger went on to illustrate how the presence of hapten inhibited enzymatic proteolysis of the IgM Fab fragment, also suggesting either a conformational change in the antibody or steric blocking by the hapten.[63] The protection of the Fab fragment from proteolysis following antigen binding was first described by another group using rabbit antibodies in 1965.[64] However, much of this early work provided only indirect evidence of conformational changes that were localized to the Fab, still failing indicate any conformational changes in the Fc. The techniques available at the time were also not sensitive enough to refute alternative explanations for the positive results.

With the application of X-ray crystallography to determining large protein structures, direct evidence of conformational changes began to appear in the literature. In 1976, Huber et al. used crystallographic and molecular modeling data to develop an allosteric model, where antigen binding was thought to trigger a conformational change that could travel from the V region along conserved residues in interchain and interdomain contacts to induce conformational changes in the Fc region.[65] These conformational changes were thought to enhance Fc receptor affinity, inhibit Fab bending, and increase whole antibody rigidity. The authors also hypothesized that the flexibility of the hinge allowed for C_{H1}-C_{H2} contacts to propagate conformational changes between the Fab and Fc. Such intramolecular signaling in antibodies, referred to as the allosteric model, was subsequently supported over the years by a number of studies. In the 1970s, Brown and Koshland described the increased fixation of complement by antigen-bound IgM, using monovalent antigens to exclude any effect from antibody cross-linking or aggregation.[66] They also validated these observations with a subsequent study showing increased accessibility of the J-chain polypeptide, which is normally folded within the terminal C_{H4} Fc domains of pentameric IgM, following exposure to both monovalent and multivalent antigens.[67] A similar observation was made by another group by measuring tryptophan fluorescence, with additional data suggesting that changes in the Fc region were dependent on the presence of interchain disulfide bonds.[68] In 1992, Horgan et al. published a study indicating that changes in the V_H region of two antibodies led to differential activation of complement.[69] The authors showed that the observation was not due to differences in affinity or avidity and suggested that V_H region changes led to different allosteric constraints on the C_H region following antigen binding. Work by Guddat et al. in 1994 provided more evidence with the fascinating observation that the addition of antigen to previously crystallized unbound Fabs resulted in the dissolution of the crystals and the formation of new crystals with different properties.[38] This indicated significant conformational changes in the Fab following antigen binding. After solving the structures of the Fab under both conditions, Guddat et al. observed significant changes in the elbow angle between the C and V domains and a large 19 Å displacement of a glutamic acid residue in the upper hinge of the heavy chain. Such a shift may have been an illustration of conformational changes propagating from the Fab to the Fc, or it may have been due to altered crystal packing. Yet, another study in 2003 used isothermal titration calorimetry (ITC) and biosensor assays to show that antigen binding inhibited interactions of the C_{H1} domain with streptococcal protein G and the C_{H2}-C_{H3} domains with staphylococcal protein A.[70] These changes were observed in IgG antibodies whose interchain disulfide linkages had been reduced. Other crystallography studies showed that antigen binding caused global changes in the quaternary structure of the V domains and illustrated that, in certain instances, V_H and V_L domains could move apart to accommodate antigen.[38,71–75] These global conformational changes, however, were not observed in all studies.[76] In 2006, another group provided experimental and theoretical evidence for an allosteric mechanism of long-distance structural changes in Fabs following antigen binding.[77] More recently, Sela-Culang et al. performed a systematic analysis of all available pairs of free and bound antibody structures, revealing many distant structural changes that occur following antigen binding.[78] Some of the observed changes included the relative orientation of the heavy and light chains, the elbow angle between the variable and constant regions, and the structure of a C_{H1} loop that forms part of the C_H-C_L interface.

Despite the later appearance of numerous positive results in the literature, most studies prior to the 1980s failed to show any conformational changes upon antigen binding. One explanation for the many inconsistencies in these results is the possibility that certain antibody germline lineages are inherently more permissive than others of conformational changes propagating from the paratope to the rest of the molecule, a prospect that will be touched on again below. Indeed, different antibody lineages may have even evolved to change their conformations in response to antigen in different ways, leading to distinct modulations of the downstream immune response. One could also speculate that different antigens binding to the same antibody may cause different conformational changes to occur, and there is some evidence for this.[66] To test these ideas, one would need to perform detailed structural analyses of many antibodies of varying germline lineages both in the presence and absence of different antigens. It is important to note that the presence of a certain conformational change does not prove a downstream function for that change, so it would also be essential to identify any differences in activation of Fc receptors, complement components, or other downstream effects.

At the same time many studies were failing to prove the existence of intramolecular signaling in antibodies, others provided evidence for an alternative mechanism by which the immune system could specifically recognize antigen-bound immunoglobulins. Demonstrations of the migration and consolidation of membrane-bound immunoglobulin receptors on lymphocyte surfaces following the addition of antigen suggested a trigger mechanism independent of conformational changes.[79,80] These data promoted an alternative hypothesis, known as the associative model, that signaling cascades upon antigen binding could be initiated by the oligomerization or cross-linking of multiple Fc receptors resulting from several antibody molecules binding to multivalent antigens. This mechanism could operate without the requirement of any structural changes in the immunoglobulin monomers themselves, relying instead on the increased avidity of numerous monomeric interactions. It also explained the prior observations of rapidly phagocytosed antibody-antigen complexes. Eventually, the importance of the associative model to antibody signaling was proven for membrane-bound Fc receptors, B cell receptors, and complement activation on antigen-bound serum immunoglobulins. As strong evidence for this signaling mechanism accumulated, the alternative hypothesis of conformational changes in antibody monomers was generally rejected, ignored, or regarded as irrelevant.[81] One reason for this lay in the wealth of negative results from studies looking for distant conformational changes following antigen binding. Those studies that did find evidence of conformational changes typically showed very small effects and the techniques were often not sophisticated enough to reject alternative explanations for the positive results. Observed conformational changes were also only rarely linked to any observable downstream effects on receptor activation. Furthermore, the elegance of the modular antibody model with separate domains evolutionarily selected to carry out distinct and independent functions was highly appealing to the increasingly reductionist landscape of science. However, given the large and increasing amount of evidence suggesting intramolecular signaling from the antibody paratope to the Fc, the allosteric model of antigen binding should be considered to play a role in antibody signaling along with the traditional model of monomer association.

6.5 CONSTANT REGION MODULATION OF ANTIBODY PROPERTIES

While most of the early research on intramolecular signaling in antibodies focused on conformational changes being transmitted from the Fab to the Fc, a number of groups beginning in the 1990s began to investigate whether conformational changes in the Fc could affect the antibody-antigen interactions in the Fab. The genesis of this research lay in the observation of unique antibody properties that were determined by the molecule's isotype. Many structural differences were immediately evident between antibodies of varying isotype, including oligomerization, molecular weight, glycosylation, interchain linkages, and molecular flexibility (Table 6.1). Over time, these structural differences were linked with many important functional properties of antibodies, including serum half-life, ability to fix complement, physical location in the body, Fc receptor affinity, and avidity for antigen.[4–6] While these diverse functional properties were generally attributed to C_H differences interacting with various components of the immune system, it was assumed that different C_H regions would not inherently affect the interaction of antibody with antigen. In 1991, Kato et al. showed that significant binding changes occurred in murine Fabs whose C_{H1} domains were switched with the homologous domains from IgG2a and IgG2b subclasses.[82] These antibody fragments possessed identical V_L, C_L, and V_H domains but exhibited differing ^{13}C NMR spectra indicating altered domain-domain interactions upon binding of the same hapten antigen. These variable-region-identical Fabs were also shown to have significant changes in the chemical shifts of the CDR-H3 loop upon antigen binding. This study by Kato et al. was an early indicator that changes in the antibody isotype could cause subtle alterations in the chemical environment of nearby V_H CDRs and even the more distant light chain domains of the Fab, ultimately yielding differences in antigen binding.

A few years later, Pritsch et al. examined the binding of IgA1 and IgG1 Fabs to antigen using surface plasmon resonance (SPR), showing significant changes in the association rate constants between the two isotypes.[83] Based on their observations, the authors suggested that antibody class switching to a different C_H could play a role in affinity maturation and contribute to an antibody's fine specificity for antigen. Their results suggested an allosteric role for the C_{H1} domain in modulating the antibody combining site. In 2000, the same group studied human IgA1 and IgG1 variable-region-identical antibodies to tubulin isolated from the serum of a lymphoma patient, finding significant differences in affinity to a common β-tubulin motif.[84] The group then cloned and expressed the IgA1 V_L and V_H domains with the C_L κ and either the C_H μ or $\gamma 1$ exons, generating complete recombinant IgM and IgG1 antibodies. They found that both the recombinant and serum IgG1 antibodies had similar K_D values on the order of 10^{-7} M, while the serum IgA1 and recombinant IgM had 14- and 43-fold higher affinities, respectively. They also showed that the increased valency of IgM and IgA could not account for the differences in observed affinity by using both Fab fragments and monomeric antibodies derived from the original IgM and IgA isotypes. Based on other antibody crystal structures, Pritsch et al. generated models of the C_{H1}-V_H interface for both IgG1 and IgA1. These models showed a striking conformational change in one of the C_{H1} loops between the two isotypes. The C_{H1} loop also had direct contacts to the V_H domain, suggesting a possible mechanism for isotype-specific allosteric modulation of the V region, and by extension antigen affinity.

In 2002, McLean et al. created a set of chimeric antibodies to the polysaccharide capsule of the pathogenic fungus *Cryptococcus neoformans*.[85] This antibody set consisted of the V_L and V_H domains of a murine precursor antibody joined to the human C_L and variants of the human C_H. All antibodies in the set possessed identical V_H, V_L, and C_L regions with varying C_H domains. The group compared IgA1, IgG1–4, and IgM isotypes of these variable-region-identical antibodies, finding differences in their fine specificities for both multivalent polysaccharide antigen and a monovalent peptide antigen mimetic. Based on immunofluorescence experiments, the group found that IgG3 and IgM isotypes bound the fungal capsule with a punctate pattern, while the other isotypes bound with an annular pattern. Earlier studies with two different antibodies to *C. neoformans* found that the annular binding pattern correlates with opsonic efficiency for phagocytosis and protective efficacy.[86] A subsequent study used SPR to show that the various chimeric antibody isotypes had differences in the kinetics and thermodynamics of antigen binding.[87] This study also indicated that glycosylation had no effect on antigen binding. Because these observations were made with human-mouse chimeric antibodies, there was concern that affinity differences could represent an effect of creating artificial antibody molecules. Torres et al. addressed this concern by using a set of completely murine isotype-switch variants of two different precursor antibodies to the *C. neoformans* capsular polysaccharide.[88] The precursor antibodies originated from different heavy and light chain germline genes and the studied subclass variants included IgG1, IgG2a, IgG2b, and IgG3. Subclass-dependent differences in the fine specificity for antigen and idiotypic properties were evident in both murine antibody families. The group later showed, using SPR and ITC, that altering the C_H region caused changes in the kinetic and thermodynamic properties of antigen binding.[89,90] These experiments used monovalent peptide antigens to probe binding by ELISA, SPR, and ITC. SPR analysis was performed with Fabs to isolate the isotype effects to the C_{H1} domain. The group found that the IgG1 Fab showed the highest binding affinity and concluded that the isotype effects were potentially only owing to structural differences in the C_{H1} domain.[89] The ITC results showed a 2:1 binding stoichiometry of the monovalent peptide with antibody monomers along with significant subclass-dependent differences in association constants.[90]

A number of other groups have published more recent studies detailing changes in antigen specificity following alteration of the C_H region. One study showed that switching an anti-HIV IgG2 to IgG1 increased reactivity to infected cells and virions, while switching to IgG3 decreased reactivity.[91] Michaelsen et al. constructed a set of variable-region-identical, human-mouse chimeric antibodies to *Neisseria meningitidis*, which were found to have differences in binding activities and functional properties.[92] Interestingly, pentameric IgM had reduced affinity compared to IgG1, indicating that its increased avidity was not enough to improve binding over the IgG1 isotype. Another group demonstrated differences in binding affinity by comparing hinge-deleted and intact antibodies. Based on this work, intact IgG1 was found to bind monovalent antigens with higher affinities than a hinge-deleted IgG1, but this difference was not observed using multivalent antigens.[93] Interestingly, IgG4 showed increased affinity following deletion of the hinge region. This study indicated that regions distal to the C_{H1} may be involved in isotype-mediated differences in specificity. It also illustrated that these specificity differences may depend on the type and valency of antigen.

Within the past decade, many more examples have been found of constant region changes affecting antibody specificity. In 2012, Tudor et al. reported increased binding affinity to an HIV-1 *env* component (glycoprotein 41) when switching a broadly neutralizing human IgG1 to an IgA2.[94] This study also noted significant changes to the epitope specificity and increases in anti-HIV-1 activity. A later report used the same antibodies to compare binding affinities of Fabs to whole IgGs via ITC, resulting in the highest affinities being observed with whole antibody.[95] This indicated that the hinge, C_{H2}, and/or C_{H3} domains also had an effect on antigen affinity. In 2013, a group studying a different antibody to HIV-1 showed that class-switching from IgG1 to IgA2 led to significant increases in affinity for the other HIV *env* product, glycoprotein 120.[96] Two recent studies by Xia et al. broadened these techniques to anti-DNA immunoglobulins, finding differences in affinity via SPR along with changes in tryptophan fluorescence and circular dichroic spectra following antigen binding.[97,98] In 2015, another group found differences in affinity, as measured by SPR, for the grass pollen allergen Phl p 7, using a panel of human IgG1–4 and IgA1–2 antibodies with identical V regions.[99] The use of similar techniques by Hovenden et al. with another set of antibodies to the *Bacillus anthracis* capsule showed that class-switching from IgG3 to IgG1, IgG2a, and IgG2b caused a reduction in binding affinity and a corresponding loss of protection.[100] Interestingly, this study showed that the lowest affinity isotype's C_{H1} domain (from IgG2b) did not reduce antigen affinity when linked to the protective isotype's C_{H2} and C_{H3} domains (from IgG3). Swapping out the IgG3 C_{H2} or C_{H3} domains, however, caused decreases in affinity with the largest effect localized to the C_{H2} region. Furthermore, deglycosylation of the IgG3 had no effect on affinity. While Fc-Fc interactions could contribute to the observed effects, the authors concluded that the C_{H2} domain plays a direct role in antibody affinity by either influencing the overall antibody charge or modifying the electrostatic environment of the paratope. Notably, this result is in contrast to earlier observations that localized isotype-mediated effects on specificity to the hinge or to the C_{H1} domain.[89,93,101,102] Hovenden et al. also observed that hinge flexibility did not correlate with antigen affinity, as had been previously hypothesized by others.[103]

One frequent explanation for the observation of isotype-specific differences in specificity is the existence of subclass-mediated differences in functional affinity. While the increased avidity of IgM and IgA multimeric isotypes had long been well characterized, studies in the late 1980s and early 1990s began to suggest differences in avidity between monomeric antibodies of differing subclasses. Greenspan et al. showed that murine IgG3 antibodies to streptococcal cell wall polysaccharide bound cooperatively and that this observation was dependent on the Fc region.[104] Subsequent studies compared the parental IgG3 to IgG1 and IgG2b switch-variants. This work showed that IgG3 bound bacterial antigens with the highest affinity and with a different binding pattern than either of the other isotypes or the IgG3 F(ab')$_2$ fragment.[105–107] One of these publications showed that the three different isotypes bound monovalent antigens with comparable affinities and that differences were only observed with multivalent antigens, consistent with the hypothesis that IgG3 exhibited cooperative binding through increased avidity.[106] Several other groups around this time reported similar results with different variable-region-identical antibody families.[103,108] Fulpius et al. showed that switching a pathogenic cryoglobulin from IgG3 to IgG1 resulted in a dramatic decrease in cryoglobulin activity.[109] Most of these studies found increased avidity in IgG3 antibodies, suggesting that a region of the $\gamma3\,C_H$ leads to the association of immunoglobulin monomers. Mechanistic support for this idea arrived with the realization that subclass-specific glycosylation sites in the C_{H3} domain are essential for the self-association of IgG3 antibodies.[10]

While the increased functional affinity associated with certain isotypes was shown to play a role in some C_H-mediated specificity changes, this theory could not explain observed differences in specificity for monovalent antigens or when Fab fragments were used instead of intact antibody. The major proposed explanation for these observations is the allosteric modification of the antibody paratope by changes in the C region structure. Many of the studies detailed earlier offer indirect support of this hypothesis, but another body of work has accumulated detailing the specific structural changes that occur following class-switching. A study by Adachi et al. used molecular dynamics simulations of several IgG1 variants (free Fab, bound Fab, and bound Fv) to show numerous structural differences in the paratope following removal of the C regions.[110] The most notable changes included the presence of 17 additional water molecules at the antibody-antigen interface and major conformational changes in the second upper loop of the C_L region. In 2010, our group showed that V and C regions are structurally coupled during antigen binding by measuring the circular dichroic spectra of a family of anticryptococcal immunoglobulins.[111] Tryptophan fluorescence, NMR, X-ray crystallography, and molecular modeling studies of these antibodies with a monovalent peptide antigen later showed isotype-dependent differences in the paratopes and elbow angles of the Fabs.[112,113] Remarkably, these studies also showed that this family of variable-region-identical antibodies is catalytic and able to hydrolyze a peptide antigen. The rates of hydrolysis and resulting peptide fragments were found to vary by isotype, strongly indicating significant changes in the antibody paratope. One study by Xia et al. that was discussed earlier used antibodies from a murine systemic lupus erythematosus model to show isotype-specific changes in secondary structure upon antigen binding along with variations in antigen-binding profiles that were ultimately linked to significant differences in renal pathogenesis and survival.[97] Another group compared crystal structures of variable-region-identical human IgA1 and IgG1 subtypes, revealing that the IgA1 possessed greater interdomain and interchain rigidity.[114] This analysis also showed a change in the elbow angle between the V_H and C_H domains, resulting in a realignment of the V_L and V_H domains that could directly cause allosteric modifications of the paratope. The group also hypothesized that rigidity differences between isotypes may lead to differences in conformational entropy and ultimately correlate with antigen affinity. Small-angle X-ray scattering experiments by two independent groups revealed significant conformational differences among various IgG subclasses.[115,116] Eryilmaz et al. proposed the idea that global isotype-specific structures are the result of cross-domain allosteric relationships between various V and C region combinations, which can dramatically impact overall antibody shape.[115] Tian et al. found significant differences in hinge angles and global conformation between the IgG subtypes, suggesting that Fab-Fab and Fab-Fc interactions are impacted by isotype.[116]

Many of the studies showing contributions of the C_H region to antibody affinity and specificity have been summarized in several review articles.[117–119] It is important to point out that a number of publications also fail to show differences in antigen affinity between variable-region-identical antibodies of differing isotype.[120–126] While these negative results may reflect insufficient sensitivity to detect isotype-dependent changes in affinity, it is also possible that certain antibodies may be more permissive than others of conformational changes in the C_H region affecting the antigen-antibody interaction. In this regard, we analyzed antibody sequences from the literature and classified them according to whether or not isotype-switch variants exhibited differences in antigen specificity.[118] The germline immunoglobulin gene for each V_H and V_L region was identified and the sequences were clustered by edit distance. This analysis showed that certain related immunoglobulin V gene families may be more associated than others with antigen specificity changes following isotype switching. Interestingly, all of the human antibodies with a λ C_L type were nonpermissive of specificity changes. To our knowledge, no detailed binding studies of variable-region-identical immunoglobulins with varying C_L domains have been performed. The combination of certain V_L and V_H lineages may be yet another variable involved in C-mediated specificity changes. This concept is similar to the idea that certain germline lineages may be inherently more permissive than others of conformational changes propagating in the opposite direction, from the paratope to the Fc. It is unclear, however, whether a germline predisposition for paratope-to-Fc intramolecular signaling would also indicate the presence of C_H-to-paratope intramolecular signaling. Indeed, detailed structural studies of antigen binding with isotype-switch variants from many more antibody germline families will be needed to test these hypotheses.

Two of the major barriers to deciphering the allosteric role of the C region in antibody-antigen interactions include the lack of a clear mechanism and the substantial variation between specific antibodies. Despite these difficulties, it has become evident over the past three decades that immunoglobulin constant regions often have a significant allosteric impact on antigen binding, supporting the view that class-switching is yet another contributor to the diversity of the antibody repertoire. We note that another major contributor to antibody diversity—somatic hypermutation—is driven by some of the same proteins involved in class-switch recombination, elegantly joining two processes that dramatically impact mature antibody specificity.[127] This conclusion also adheres nicely to the theory of antibody multispecificity, where a single immunoglobulin can adopt multiple conformations with varying antigen specificities.[128] This may reflect an ancient principle of evolution, enabling a limited set of protein sequences to carry out multiple functions.[129] The implications of C-mediated effects on specificity extend to many areas of immunology, including primary and secondary B cell responses, idiotype reactivity, and vaccine development. Observations that class-switching can result in reactivity to self-antigens have extensive implications for autoimmune conditions.[98] Furthermore, moving toward a mechanistic understanding of C_H-mediated changes in affinity has the potential to dramatically impact the field of antibody engineering and the design of therapeutic monoclonal antibodies.[130]

6.6 CONCLUDING REMARKS

Many early studies deciphering the structure and function of the immunoglobulin molecule provided great strides in our understanding of immunology. The ability to make such leaps of knowledge was frequently enabled by the modular nature of the molecule, as scientists were able to dissociate and digest peptide chains to link specific functions to specific parts of the antibody. While this conception of the antibody molecule proved illuminating and transformed our understanding of immunology, it was also an oversimplification of the structural nuances that determine an antibody's fine specificity. Substantial evidence indicates that an immunoglobulin's V and C domains are not functionally independent and that allosteric effects can propagate between the different domains of the molecule. A large body of work had shown C region conformational changes following antigen binding, but it is still not clear whether this reliably impacts antibody effector functions. Long-distance conformational changes, however, have been shown to affect antibody-antigen interactions and global antibody structure. It is now clear that the C region plays a major role in antigen binding and is a contributor to antibody diversity. Determining how conformational changes are propagated through the molecule is difficult because the mechanism seems to involve a complex network of interdomain and interchain contacts that may vary with different C_H, C_L, V_H, and V_L combinations. Intramolecular interactions between the H and L chains and the V and C domains, along with variations in the hinge and elbow angle, all play an essential role in modifying the paratope and its fine specificity for antigen. The C_{H1} domain, in particular, seems to be a linchpin of this network, transmitting structural changes between its contacts to the C_L, V_H, and hinge region. As future studies focus on identifying the structural determinants of intramolecular signaling in antibodies, we will transition to a new model of antibody structure that better captures the complex and important roles these fascinating molecules play in the immune system.

REFERENCES

1. von Behring E, Kitasato S. The mechanism of immunity in animals to diptheria and tetanus. *Dtsch Med Wochenschr* 1890;**16**:1113–4.
2. Tiselius A, Kabat EA. An electrophoretic study of immune sera and purified antibody preparations. *J Exp Med* 1939;**69**(1):119–31.
3. Harris LJ, Skaletsky E, McPherson A. Crystallographic structure of an intact IgG1 monoclonal antibody. *J Mol Biol* 1998;**275**(5):861–72.
4. Nezlin RS. *The immunoglobulins: structure and function.* xiii. San Diego: Academic Press; 1998269.

5. Schroeder Jr. HW, Cavacini L. Structure and function of immunoglobulins. *J Allergy Clin Immunol* 2010;**125**(2 Suppl. 2):S41–52.

6. Nisonoff A, Hopper JE, Spring SB. *The antibody molecule.* xiv. New York: Academic Press; 1975542.

7. Arnold JN, Wormald MR, Sim RB, Rudd PM, Dwek RA. The impact of glycosylation on the biological function and structure of human immunoglobulins. *Annu Rev Immunol* 2007;**25**:21–50.

8. Radaev S, Sun PD. Recognition of IgG by Fcgamma receptor. The role of Fc glycosylation and the binding of peptide inhibitors. *J Biol Chem* 2001;**276**(19):16478–83.

9. Butler M, Quelhas D, Critchley AJ, Carchon H, Hebestreit HF, Hibbert RG, et al. Detailed glycan analysis of serum glycoproteins of patients with congenital disorders of glycosylation indicates the specific defective glycan processing step and provides an insight into pathogenesis. *Glycobiology* 2003;**13**(9):601–22.

10. Panka DJ. Glycosylation is influential in murine IgG3 self-association. *Mol Immunol* 1997;**34**(8–9):593–8.

11. Wallick SC, Kabat EA, Morrison SL. Glycosylation of a VH residue of a monoclonal antibody against alpha (1–6) dextran increases its affinity for antigen. *J Exp Med* 1988;**168**(3):1099–109.

12. Frenzel A, Hust M, Schirrmann T. Expression of recombinant antibodies. *Front Immunol* 2013;**4**:217.

13. Hamers-Casterman C, Atarhouch T, Muyldermans S, Robinson G, Hamers C, Songa EB, et al. Naturally occurring antibodies devoid of light chains. *Nature* 1993;**363**(6428):446–8.

14. Roux KH, Greenberg AS, Greene L, Strelets L, Avila D, McKinney EC, et al. Structural analysis of the nurse shark (new) antigen receptor (NAR): molecular convergence of NAR and unusual mammalian immunoglobulins. *Proc Natl Acad Sci U S A* 1998;**95**(20):11804–9.

15. Feng M, Gao W, Wang R, Chen W, Man YG, Figg WD, et al. Therapeutically targeting glypican-3 via a conformation-specific single-domain antibody in hepatocellular carcinoma. *Proc Natl Acad Sci U S A* 2013;**110**(12):E1083–91.

16. Cossins AJ, Harrison S, Popplewell AG, Gore MG. Recombinant production of a VL single domain antibody in Escherichia coli and analysis of its interaction with peptostreptococcal protein L. *Protein Expr Purif* 2007;**51**(2):253–9.

17. Porter RR. The formation of a specific inhibitor by hydrolysis of rabbit antiovalbumin. *Biochem J* 1950;**46**(4):479–84.

18. Porter RR. The hydrolysis of rabbit y-globulin and antibodies with crystalline papain. *Biochem J* 1959;**73**:119–26.

19. Edelman GM, Poulik MD. Studies on structural units of the gamma-globulins. *J Exp Med* 1961;**113**:861–84.

20. Edelman GM, Cunningham BA, Gall WE, Gottlieb PD, Rutishauser U, Waxdal MJ. The covalent structure of an entire gammaG immunoglobulin molecule. *Proc Natl Acad Sci U S A* 1969;**63**(1):78–85.

21. Wu TT, Kabat EA. An analysis of the sequences of the variable regions of Bence Jones proteins and myeloma light chains and their implications for antibody complementarity. *J Exp Med* 1970;**132**(2):211–50.

22. Kabat EA, Wu TT. Attempts to locate complementarity-determining residues in the variable positions of light and heavy chains. *Ann N Y Acad Sci* 1971;**190**:382–93.

23. Kabat EA, Wu TT, Bilofsky H. Unusual distributions of amino acids in complementarity-determining (hypervariable) segments of heavy and light chains of immunoglobulins and their possible roles in specificity of antibody-combining sites. *J Biol Chem* 1977;**252**(19):6609–16.

24. Tonegawa S, Steinberg C, Dube S, Bernardini A. Evidence for somatic generation of antibody diversity. *Proc Natl Acad Sci U S A* 1974;**71**(10):4027–31.

25. Tonegawa S. Reiteration frequency of immunoglobulin light chain genes: further evidence for somatic generation of antibody diversity. *Proc Natl Acad Sci U S A* 1976;**73**(1):203–7.

26. Hozumi N, Tonegawa S. Evidence for somatic rearrangement of immunoglobulin genes coding for variable and constant regions. *Proc Natl Acad Sci U S A* 1976;**73**(10):3628–32.

27. Brack C, Hirama M, Lenhard-Schuller R, Tonegawa S. A complete immunoglobulin gene is created by somatic recombination. *Cell* 1978;**15**(1):1–14.

28. Davis MM, Calame K, Early PW, Livant DL, Joho R, Weissman IL, et al. An immunoglobulin heavy-chain gene is formed by at least two recombinational events. *Nature* 1980;**283**(5749):733–9.

29. Early P, Huang H, Davis M, Calame K, Hood L. An immunoglobulin heavy chain variable region gene is generated from three segments of DNA: VH, D and JH. *Cell* 1980;**19**(4):981–92.

30. Maki R, Traunecker A, Sakano H, Roeder W, Tonegawa S. Exon shuffling generates an immunoglobulin heavy chain gene. *Proc Natl Acad Sci U S A* 1980;**77**(4):2138–42.

31. Davies DR, Padlan EA, Segal DM. Three-dimensional structure of immunoglobulins. *Annu Rev Biochem* 1975;**44**:639–67.

32. Padlan EA, Davies DR. Variability of three-dimensional structure in immunoglobulins. *Proc Natl Acad Sci U S A* 1975;**72**(3):819–23.

33. Harris LJ, Larson SB, Hasel KW, McPherson A. Refined structure of an intact IgG2a monoclonal antibody. *Biochemistry* 1997;**36**(7):1581–97.

34. Colman PM. Structure of antibody-antigen complexes: implications for immune recognition. *Adv Immunol* 1988;**43**:99–132.

35. Rini JM, Schulze-Gahmen U, Wilson IA. Structural evidence for induced fit as a mechanism for antibody-antigen recognition. *Science* 1992;**255**(5047):959–65.

36. Schulze-Gahmen U, Rini JM, Wilson IA. Detailed analysis of the free and bound conformations of an antibody. X-ray structures of Fab 17/9 and three different Fab-peptide complexes. *J Mol Biol* 1993;**234**(4):1098–118.

37. Bizebard T, Gigant B, Rigolet P, Rasmussen B, Diat O, Bosecke P, et al. Structure of influenza virus haemagglutinin complexed with a neutralizing antibody. *Nature* 1995;**376**(6535):92–4.

38. Guddat LW, Shan L, Anchin JM, Linthicum DS, Edmundson AB. Local and transmitted conformational changes on complexation of an anti-sweetener Fab. *J Mol Biol* 1994;**236**(1):247–74.

39. Scherf T, Hiller R, Anglister J. NMR observation of interactions in the combining site region of an antibody using a spin-labeled peptide antigen and NOESY difference spectroscopy. *FASEB J* 1995;**9**(1):120–6.

40. Sheriff S, Chang CY, Jeffrey PD, Bajorath J. X-ray structure of the uncomplexed anti-tumor antibody BR96 and comparison with its antigen-bound form. *J Mol Biol* 1996;**259**(5):938–46.

41. Lescar J, Stouracova R, Riottot MM, Chitarra V, Brynda J, Fabry M, et al. Three-dimensional structure of an Fab-peptide complex: structural basis of HIV-1 protease inhibition by a monoclonal antibody. *J Mol Biol* 1997;**267**(5):1207–22.

42. Benacerraf B, Sebestyen M, Cooper NS. The clearance of antigen antibody complexes from the blood by the reticuloendothelial system. *J Immunol* 1959;**82**(2):131–7.

43. Shinomiya T, Koyama J. In vitro uptake and digestion of immune complexes containing guinea-pig IgG1 and IgG2 antibodies by macrophages. *Immunology* 1976;**30**(2):267–75.

44. Stryer L. Implications of X-ray crystallographic studies of protein structure. *Annu Rev Biochem* 1968;**37**:25–50.

45. Stryer L, Griffith OH. A spin-labeled hapten. *Proc Natl Acad Sci U S A* 1965;**54**(6):1785–91.

46. Yguerabide J, Epstein HF, Stryer L. Segmental flexibility in an antibody molecule. *J Mol Biol* 1970;**51**(3):573–90.

47. Werner TC, Bunting JR, Cathou RE. The shape of immunoglobulin G molecules in solution. *Proc Natl Acad Sci U S A* 1972;**69**(4):795–9.

48. Segal DM, Padlan EA, Cohen GH, Rudikoff S, Potter M, Davies DR. The three-dimensional structure of a phosphorylcholine-binding mouse immunoglobulin Fab and the nature of the antigen binding site. *Proc Natl Acad Sci U S A* 1974;**71**(11):4298–302.

49. Steiner LA, Lowey S. Optical rotatory dispersion studies of rabbit gamma-G-immunoglobulin and its papain fragments. *J Biol Chem* 1966;**241**(1):231–40.

50. Cathou RE, Kulczycki Jr. A, Haber E. Structural features of gamma-immunoglobulin, antibody, and their fragments. Circular dichroism studies. *Biochemistry* 1968;**7**(11):3958–64.

51. Ishizaka K, Campbell DH. Biologic activity of soluble antigen-antibody complexes. V. Change of optical rotation by the formation of skin reactive complexes. *J Immunol* 1959;**83**:318–26.

52. Metzger H. The antigen receptor problem. *Annu Rev Biochem* 1970;**39**:889–928.

53. Feinstein A, Rowe AJ. Molecular mechanism of formation of an antigen-antibody complex. *Nature* 1965;**205**:147–9.

54. Valentine RC, Green NM. Electron microscopy of an antibody-hapten complex. *J Mol Biol* 1967;**27**(3):615–7.

55. Oi VT, Vuong TM, Hardy R, Reidler J, Dangle J, Herzenberg LA, et al. Correlation between segmental flexibility and effector function of antibodies. *Nature* 1984;**307**(5947):136–40.

56. Saphire EO, Stanfield RL, Crispin MD, Parren PW, Rudd PM, Dwek RA, et al. Contrasting IgG structures reveal extreme asymmetry and flexibility. *J Mol Biol* 2002;**319**(1):9–18.

57. Nisonoff A, Wissler FC, Woernley DL. Properties of univalent fragments of rabbit antibody isolated by specific adsorption. *Arch Biochem Biophys* 1960;**88**:241–9.

58. Velick SF, Parker CW, Eisen HN. Excitation energy transfer and the quantitative study of the antibody Hapten reaction. *Proc Natl Acad Sci U S A* 1960;**46**(11):1470–82.

59. Ashman RF, Metzger H. A waldenstrom macroglobulin which binds nitrophenyl ligands. *J Biol Chem* 1969;**244**(12):3405–14.

60. Holowka DA, Strosberg AD, Kimball JW, Haber E, Cathou RE. Changes in intrinsic circular dichroism of several homogeneous anti-type 3 pneumococcal antibodies on binding of a small hapten. *Proc Natl Acad Sci U S A* 1972;**69**(11):3399–403.

61. Warner C, Schumaker V, Karush F. The detection of a conformational change in the antibody molecule upon interaction with hapten. *Biochem Biophys Res Commun* 1970;**38**(1):125–8.

62. Ashman RF, Kaplan AP, Metzger H. A search for conformational change on ligand binding in a human M macroglobulin. I. Circular dichroism and hydrogen exchange. *Immunochemistry* 1971;**8**(7):627–41.

63. Ashman RF, Metzger H. A search for conformational change on ligand binding in a human M macroglobulin. II. Susceptibility to proteolysis. *Immunochemistry* 1971;**8**(7):643–56.

64. Grossberg AL, Markus G, Pressman D. Change in antibody conformation induced by hapten. *Proc Natl Acad Sci U S A* 1965;**54**(3):942–5.

65. Huber R, Deisenhofer J, Colman PM, Matsushima M, Palm W. Crystallographic structure studies of an IgG molecule and an Fc fragment. *Nature* 1976;**264**(5585):415–20.

66. Brown JC, Koshland ME. Activation of antibody Fc function by antigen-induced conformational changes. *Proc Natl Acad Sci U S A* 1975;**72**(12):5111–5.

67. Brown JC, Koshland ME. Evidence for a long-range conformational change induced by antigen binding to IgM antibody. *Proc Natl Acad Sci U S A* 1977;**74**(12):5682–6.

68. Schlessinger J, Steinberg IZ, Givol D, Hochman J, Pecht I. Antigen-induced conformational changes in antibodies and their Fab fragments studied by circular polarization of fluorescence. *Proc Natl Acad Sci U S A* 1975;**72**(7):2775–9.

69. Horgan C, Brown K, Pincus SH. Effect of H chain V region on complement activation by immobilized immune complexes. *J Immunol* 1992;**149**(1):127–35.

70. Oda M, Kozono H, Morii H, Azuma T. Evidence of allosteric conformational changes in the antibody constant region upon antigen binding. *Int Immunol* 2003;**15**(3):417–26.

71. Bhat TN, Bentley GA, Fischmann TO, Boulot G, Poljak RJ. Small rearrangements in structures of Fv and Fab fragments of antibody D1.3 on antigen binding. *Nature* 1990;**347**(6292):483–5.

72. Herron JN, He XM, Ballard DW, Blier PR, Pace PE, Bothwell AL, et al. An autoantibody to single-stranded DNA: comparison of the three-dimensional structures of the unliganded Fab and a deoxynucleotide-Fab complex. *Proteins* 1991;**11**(3):159–75.

73. Stanfield RL, Takimoto-Kamimura M, Rini JM, Profy AT, Wilson IA. Major antigen-induced domain rearrangements in an antibody. *Structure* 1993;**1**(2):83–93.

74. Tormo J, Blaas D, Parry NR, Rowlands D, Stuart D, Fita I. Crystal structure of a human rhinovirus neutralizing antibody complexed with a peptide derived from viral capsid protein VP2. *EMBO J* 1994;**13**(10):2247–56.

75. Guddat LW, Shan L, Fan ZC, Andersen KN, Rosauer R, Linthicum DS, et al. Intramolecular signaling upon complexation. *FASEB J* 1995;**9**(1):101–6.

76. Jeffrey PD, Strong RK, Sieker LC, Chang CY, Campbell RL, Petsko GA, et al. 26-10 Fab-digoxin complex: affinity and specificity due to surface complementarity. *Proc Natl Acad Sci U S A* 1993;**90**(21):10310–4.

77. Piekarska B, Drozd A, Konieczny L, Krol M, Jurkowski W, Roterman I, et al. The indirect generation of long-distance structural changes in antibodies upon their binding to antigen. *Chem Biol Drug Des* 2006;**68**(5):276–83.

78. Sela-Culang I, Alon S, Ofran Y. A systematic comparison of free and bound antibodies reveals binding-related conformational changes. *J Immunol* 2012;**189**(10):4890–9.

79. Dunham EK, Unanue ER, Benacerraf B. Antigen binding and capping by lymphocytes of genetic nonresponder mice. *J Exp Med* 1972;**136**(2):403–8.

80. Loor F, Forni L, Pernis B. The dynamic state of the lymphocyte membrane. Factors affecting the distribution and turnover of surface immunoglobulins. *Eur J Immunol* 1972;**2**(3):203–12.

81. Metzger H. Effect of antigen binding on the properties of antibody. *Adv Immunol* 1974;**18**:169–207.

82. Kato K, Matsunaga C, Odaka A, Yamato S, Takaha W, Shimada I, et al. Carbon-13 NMR study of switch variant anti-dansyl antibodies: antigen binding and domain-domain interactions. *Biochemistry* 1991;**30**(26):6604–10.

83. Pritsch O, Hudry-Clergeon G, Buckle M, Petillot Y, Bouvet JP, Gagnon J, et al. Can immunoglobulin C(H)1 constant region domain modulate antigen binding affinity of antibodies? *J Clin Invest* 1996;**98**(10):2235–43.

84. Pritsch O, Magnac C, Dumas G, Bouvet JP, Alzari P, Dighiero G. Can isotype switch modulate antigen-binding affinity and influence clonal selection? *Eur J Immunol* 2000;**30**(12):3387–95.

85. McLean GR, Torres M, Elguezabal N, Nakouzi A, Casadevall A. Isotype can affect the fine specificity of an antibody for a polysaccharide antigen. *J Immunol* 2002;**169**(3):1379–86.

86. Nussbaum G, Cleare W, Casadevall A, Scharff MD, Valadon P. Epitope location in the Cryptococcus neoformans capsule is a determinant of antibody efficacy. *J Exp Med* 1997;**185**(4):685–94.

87. Torres M, Fernandez-Fuentes N, Fiser A, Casadevall A. Exchanging murine and human immunoglobulin constant chains affects the kinetics and thermodynamics of antigen binding and chimeric antibody autoreactivity. *PLoS One* 2007;**2**(12):e1310.

88. Torres M, May R, Scharff MD, Casadevall A. Variable-region-identical antibodies differing in isotype demonstrate differences in fine specificity and idiotype. *J Immunol* 2005;**174**(4):2132–42.

89. Torres M, Fernandez-Fuentes N, Fiser A, Casadevall A. The immunoglobulin heavy chain constant region affects kinetic and thermodynamic parameters of antibody variable region interactions with antigen. *J Biol Chem* 2007;**282**(18):13917–27.

90. Dam TK, Torres M, Brewer CF, Casadevall A. Isothermal titration calorimetry reveals differential binding thermodynamics of variable region-identical antibodies differing in constant region for a univalent ligand. *J Biol Chem* 2008;**283**(46):31366–70.

91. Liu F, Bergami PL, Duval M, Kuhrt D, Posner M, Cavacini L. Expression and functional activity of isotype and subclass switched human monoclonal antibody reactive with the base of the V3 loop of HIV-1 gp120. *AIDS Res Hum Retrovir* 2003;**19**(7):597–607.

92. Michaelsen TE, Ihle O, Beckstrom KJ, Herstad TK, Sandin RH, Kolberg J, et al. Binding properties and anti-bacterial activities of V-region identical, human IgG and IgM antibodies, against group B Neisseria meningitidis. *Biochem Soc Trans* 2003;**31**(Pt 5):1032–5.

93. Horgan C, Brown K, Pincus SH. Studies on antigen binding by intact and hinge-deleted chimeric antibodies. *J Immunol* 1993;**150**(12):5400–7.

94. Tudor D, Yu H, Maupetit J, Drillet AS, Bouceba T, Schwartz-Cornil I, et al. Isotype modulates epitope specificity, affinity, and antiviral activities of anti-HIV-1 human broadly neutralizing 2F5 antibody. *Proc Natl Acad Sci U S A* 2012;**109**(31):12680–5.

95. Crespillo S, Casares S, Mateo PL, Conejero-Lara F. Thermodynamic analysis of the binding of 2F5 (Fab and immunoglobulin G forms) to its gp41 epitope reveals a strong influence of the immunoglobulin Fc region on affinity. *J Biol Chem* 2014;**289**(2):594–9.

96. Tomaras GD, Ferrari G, Shen X, Alam SM, Liao HX, Pollara J, et al. Vaccine-induced plasma IgA specific for the C1 region of the HIV-1 envelope blocks binding and effector function of IgG. *Proc Natl Acad Sci U S A* 2013;**110**(22):9019–24.

97. Xia Y, Janda A, Eryilmaz E, Casadevall A, Putterman C. The constant region affects antigen binding of antibodies to DNA by altering secondary structure. *Mol Immunol* 2013;**56**(1–2):28–37.

98. Xia Y, Pawar RD, Nakouzi AS, Herlitz L, Broder A, Liu K, et al. The constant region contributes to the antigenic specificity and renal pathogenicity of murine anti-DNA antibodies. *J Autoimmun* 2012;**39**(4):398–411.

99. Dodev TS, Bowen H, Shamji MH, Bax HJ, Beavil AJ, McDonnell JM, et al. Inhibition of allergen-dependent IgE activity by antibodies of the same specificity but different class. *Allergy* 2015;**70**(6):720–4.

100. Hovenden M, Hubbard MA, Aucoin DP, Thorkildson P, Reed DE, Welch WH, et al. IgG subclass and heavy chain domains contribute to binding and protection by mAbs to the poly gamma-D-glutamic acid capsular antigen of Bacillus anthracis. *PLoS Pathog* 2013;**9**(4):e1003306.

101. Yuan R, Casadevall A, Spira G, Scharff MD. Isotype switching from IgG3 to IgG1 converts a nonprotective murine antibody to Cryptococcus neoformans into a protective antibody. *J Immunol* 1995;**154**(4):1810–6.

102. Yuan RR, Spira G, Oh J, Paizi M, Casadevall A, Scharff MD. Isotype switching increases efficacy of antibody protection against Cryptococcus neoformans infection in mice. *Infect Immun* 1998;**66**(3):1057–62.

103. Morelock MM, Rothlein R, Bright SM, Robinson MK, Graham ET, Sabo JP, et al. Isotype choice for chimeric antibodies affects binding properties. *J Biol Chem* 1994;**269**(17):13048–55.

104. Greenspan NS, Monafo WJ, Davie JM. Interaction of IgG3 anti-streptococcal group A carbo-hydrate (GAC) antibody with streptococcal group A vaccine: enhancing and inhibiting effects of anti-GAC, anti-isotypic, and anti-idiotypic antibodies. *J Immunol* 1987;**138**(1):285–92.

105. Cooper LJ, Schimenti JC, Glass DD, Greenspan NS. H chain C domains influence the strength of binding of IgG for streptococcal group A carbohydrate. *J Immunol* 1991;**146**(8):2659–63.

106. Cooper LJ, Shikhman AR, Glass DD, Kangisser D, Cunningham MW, Greenspan NS. Role of heavy chain constant domains in antibody-antigen interaction. Apparent specificity differ-ences among streptococcal IgG antibodies expressing identical variable domains. *J Immunol* 1993;**150**(6):2231–42.

107. Cooper LJ, Robertson D, Granzow R, Greenspan NS. Variable domain-identical antibodies exhibit IgG subclass-related differences in affinity and kinetic constants as determined by surface plasmon resonance. *Mol Immunol* 1994;**31**(8):577–84.

108. Schreiber JR, Cooper LJ, Diehn S, Dahlhauser PA, Tosi MF, Glass DD, et al. Variable region-identical monoclonal antibodies of different IgG subclass directed to Pseudomo-nas aeruginosa lipopolysaccharide O-specific side chain function differently. *J Infect Dis* 1993;**167**(1):221–6.

109. Fulpius T, Spertini F, Reininger L, Izui S. Immunoglobulin heavy chain constant region de-termines the pathogenicity and the antigen-binding activity of rheumatoid factor. *Proc Natl Acad Sci U S A* 1993;**90**(6):2345–9.

110. Adachi M, Kurihara Y, Nojima H, Takeda-Shitaka M, Kamiya K, Umeyama H. Interaction between the antigen and antibody is controlled by the constant domains: normal mode dy-namics of the HEL-HyHEL-10 complex. *Protein Sci* 2003;**12**(10):2125–31.

111. Janda A, Casadevall A. Circular dichroism reveals evidence of coupling between immu-noglobulin constant and variable region secondary structure. *Mol Immunol* 2010;**47**(7–8): 1421–5.

112. Janda A, Eryilmaz E, Nakouzi A, Cowburn D, Casadevall A. Variable region identi-cal immunoglobulins differing in isotype express different paratopes. *J Biol Chem* 2012;**287**(42):35409–17.

113. Janda A, Eryilmaz E, Nakouzi A, Pohl MA, Bowen A, Casadevall A. Variable region identi-cal IgA and IgE to Cryptococcus neoformans capsular polysaccharide manifest specificity differences. *J Biol Chem* 2015;**290**(19):12090–100.

114. Correa A, Trajtenberg F, Obal G, Pritsch O, Dighiero G, Oppezzo P, et al. Structure of a human IgA1 Fab fragment at 1.55 A resolution: potential effect of the constant domains on antigen-affinity modulation. *Acta Crystallogr D Biol Crystallogr* 2013;**69**(Pt 3):388–97.

115. Eryilmaz E, Janda A, Kim J, Cordero RJ, Cowburn D, Casadevall A. Global structures of IgG isotypes expressing identical variable regions. *Mol Immunol* 2013;**56**(4):588–98.

116. Tian X, Vestergaard B, Thorolfsson M, Yang Z, Rasmussen HB, Langkilde AE. In-depth analy-sis of subclass-specific conformational preferences of IgG antibodies. *IUCrJ* 2015;**2**(Pt 1):9–18.

117. Torres M, Casadevall A. The immunoglobulin constant region contributes to affinity and specificity. *Trends Immunol* 2008;**29**(2):91–7.

118. Janda A, Bowen A, Greenspan NS, Casadevall A. Ig constant region effects on variable region structure and function. *Front Microbiol* 2016;**7**:22.

119. Sela-Culang I, Kunik V, Ofran Y. The structural basis of antibody-antigen recognition. *Front Immunol* 2013;**4**:302.

120. Adame-Gallegos JR, Shi J, McIntosh RS, Pleass RJ. The generation and evaluation of two panels of epitope-matched mouse IgG1, IgG2a, IgG2b and IgG3 antibodies specific for Plas-modium falciparum and Plasmodium yoelii merozoite surface protein 1-19 (MSP1(19)). *Exp Parasitol* 2012;**130**(4):384–93.

121. Pollack M, Koles NL, Preston MJ, Brown BJ, Pier GB. Functional properties of isotype-switched immunoglobulin M (IgM) and IgG monoclonal antibodies to Pseudomonas aeruginosa lipopolysaccharide. *Infect Immun* 1995;**63**(11):4481–8.

122. Cavacini LA, Emes CL, Wisnewski AV, Power J, Lewis G, Montefiori D, et al. Functional and molecular characterization of human monoclonal antibody reactive with the immunodominant region of HIV type 1 glycoprotein 41. *AIDS Res Hum Retrovir* 1998;**14**(14):1271–80.

123. Kelly-Quintos C, Cavacini LA, Posner MR, Goldmann D, Pier GB. Characterization of the opsonic and protective activity against Staphylococcus aureus of fully human monoclonal antibodies specific for the bacterial surface polysaccharide poly-N-acetylglucosamine. *Infect Immun* 2006;**74**(5):2742–50.

124. Porter RR. The isolation and properties of a fragment of bovine-serum albumin which retains the ability to combine with rabbit antiserum. *Biochem J* 1957;**66**(4):677–86.

125. Zaghouani H, Bonilla FA, Meek K, Bona C. Molecular basis for expression of the A48 regulatory idiotope on antibodies encoded by immunoglobulin variable-region genes from various families. *Proc Natl Acad Sci U S A* 1989;**86**(7):2341–5.

126. French HD, Porter RW, Cavanaugh EB, Longmire RL. Experimental gastroduodenal lesions induced by stimulation of the brain. *Psychosom Med* 1957;**19**(3):209–20.

127. Durandy A. Activation-induced cytidine deaminase: a dual role in class-switch recombination and somatic hypermutation. *Eur J Immunol* 2003;**33**(8):2069–73.

128. James LC, Roversi P, Tawfik DS. Antibody multispecificity mediated by conformational diversity. *Science* 2003;**299**(5611):1362–7.

129. James LC, Tawfik DS. Conformational diversity and protein evolution—a 60-year-old hypothesis revisited. *Trends Biochem Sci* 2003;**28**(7):361–8.

130. Nosanchuk JD. The interdependence of antibody C and V regions on specificity and affinity: significant implications for the engineering of therapeutic antibodies. *Virulence* 2013;**4**(6):439–40.

Index

Note: Page numbers followed by *f* indicate figures, and *t* indicate tables.

A

Abzyme, 134
Adhesion molecule
  cell-cell recognition, CD2 family proteins
    CD2-CD48 interaction, 41
    CD2/CD58 interaction, 42
    CD48 d1, 52–54
    CD58 d1, 50–52
    human sCD2, 46–48
    ligand-binding, charged residues role in,
      48–50
    rsCD2, 42–46
  immunological synapses
    CRTAM, 9
    definition, 5
    LFA-1-ICAM-1 interaction, 5–6
    nectins, 9
    SLAM family members, 5–7
Affinity-linked oligonucleotide nuclease assay
  (ALONA), 135
Allosteric antibody model, 155–156
ALWPPNLHAWVP (ALW) peptide, 135–138
Antibody-antigen interactions, constant region
  immunoglobulin molecule
    antibody isotypes, 146–149, 148*t*
    glycosylation, 149–150
    H and L chains, 146, 147*f*, 149–151
    modular antibody model, 151–154
   intramolecular signaling, 154–157
   isotype-switching, 157–163
Anti-dsDNA antibodies, SLE
  antigenic specificity and renal pathogenicity,
    130–131
  antigen recognition, features of, 129–130
  catalytic properties of, 134–136
  DNA-mimicking peptides, 136–138
  lupus nephritis, 127–128
  novel therapeutic approaches, 138–140
  structural analysis, 131–134
Antitoxin, 145–146
ASPVTARVLWKASHV peptide, 137–138
Atherosclerosis, 8–9

B

B-cell antigen receptors, 39–40
Bence-Jones proteins, 39–40
Bispecific antibody, 82

C

Catalytic antibody, 134–136
Catmab. *See* Abzyme
CD2
  CD2-CD58/48 interactions, 6–7, 11–13, 41–42
  CD48 d1, 52–54
  CD58 d1, 50–52
  human sCD2, 46–48
  ligand-binding, charged residues role in, 48–50
  rsCD2, 42–46
CD4, 9–10
CD8, 9–10
CD27, 8
CD28, 7–8
  511A1 antibody fab, 61–64
  B7-1 and B7-2, CTLA-4, 54–55
  CTLA-4/sB7-1 complex, 59–61
  CTLA-4 structure, 64–66
  sB7-1, 56–59
CD40, 8–9
CD45, 10–11, 14
CD134, 8–9
CD137, 8–9
CD357, 8–9
CDRs. *See* Complementarity-determining
    regions (CDRs)
Cell-cell recognition, 69–72
  adhesion molecule, CD2 family proteins
    CD2-CD48 interaction, 41
    CD2/CD58 interaction, 42
    CD48 d1, 52–54
    CD58 d1, 50–52
    human sCD2, 46–48
    ligand-binding, charged residues role in,
      48–50
    rsCD2, 42–46

Cell-cell recognition *(Continued)*
  costimulatory receptor, CD28-related
    proteins
      511A1 antibody fab, 61–64
      B7-1 and B7-2, CTLA-4, 54–55
      CTLA-4/sB7-1 complex, 59–61
      CTLA-4 structure, 64–66
      sB7-1, 56–59
    PD-1/ligand interactions, 66–69
Central supramolecular activation cluster
  (cSMAC), 2, 3*f*
Checkpoint receptors, 7–8
Chimeric antibody, 158–159
Class-I MHC-restricted T-cell-associated
  molecule (CRTAM), 9
CLEC. *See* C-type lectin receptor (CLEC)
Complementarity-determining regions (CDRs),
  83–85, 83*f*, 132–133, 149
Costimulatory receptors
  cell-cell recognition, CD28-related proteins
    511A1 antibody fab, 61–64
    B7-1 and B7-2, CTLA-4, 54–55
    CTLA-4/sB7-1 complex, 59–61
    CTLA-4 structure, 64–66
    sB7-1, 56–59
  immunological synapses
    CD27, 8
    CD28, 7–8
    ICOS, 8–9
Cross-reactive antibodies, 92, 93*f*
Crystallography, 40–41
C-terminal Src kinase (CSK), 10–11
C-type lectin receptor (CLEC), 115–116, 116*f*
Cysteine, 84–85
Cytoskeletal networks, 14–16
Cytotoxic T cells, 23–24
Cytotoxic T lymphocyte antigen-4 (CTLA-4),
  7–8
  B7-1 and B7-2, 54–55
  CTLA-4/sB7-1 complex, 59–61
  structure, 64–66

D

Distal supramolecular activation cluster
  (dSMAC), 2, 3*f*
DNA-catalyzing antibodies, 134
DNA-mimicking peptides, 136–138
Double-stranded DNA (dsDNA) antibodies,
  127–128
DWEYS peptide, 136, 138–139
DWEYSVWLSN peptide, 136–138

E

E-cadherin, 114, 115*f*
Ectosomes, 22–23
Endosomal sorting complexes required for the
  transport (ESCRT) system, 22–23, 23*f*
Epstein-Barr virus (EBV) infection, 8
Exocytosis, 22–24
Exosomes, 22–23
Extracellular vesicles, 22–23

F

Fc receptors, 153–154, 156–157
Filamentous actin (F-actin), 2–3, 3*f*, 14–15
FISLE-412, 138–139

G

Giant unilamellar vesicles (GUVs), 13
Glycoproteins, 40–41

H

Human cytomegalovirus (HCMV), 108–110,
  110*f*
Hybridoma technology, 81–82, 94

I

ICOS. *See* Inducible T-cell co-stimulator
  (ICOS)
IgA antibody, 146–149, 148*t*, 158
IgD antibody, 146–149, 148*t*
IgE antibody, 146–149, 148*t*
IgM antibody, 146–149, 158–159
Immunoglobulin new-antigen receptor
  (IgNAR), 150
Immunological kinapses. *See also*
  Immunological synapses
  microclusters, 2–3
  SMACs, 2–3, 3*f*
Immunological synapses
  adhesion molecules
    CRTAM, 9
    definition, 5
    LFA-1-ICAM-1 interaction, 5–6
    nectins, 9
    SLAM family members, 5–7
  characteristics of, 21
  coreceptors and transmembrane
    phosphatases, 9–11
  costimulatory and checkpoint receptors
    CD27, 8

CD28, 7–8
  CTLA-4 and PD-1, 7–8
  ICOS, 8–9
definition, 2
function of, 2
microclusters, 2–3
microvilli/filopodia
  cortical actin network, 18
  Jurkat and primary T cells, 18–19
  LFA-1-ICAM-1-mediated adhesion, 17
  nonpolarized lymphocytes, 16–17
  podosomes, 17–18
  rosette-shaped F-actin network, 19–20
  TCR and L-selection localization, 16–17
  TCR microcluster formation, 16–17
multifocal synapses, 2–3
phase separation
  cell-cell interfaces, adhesion plane of, 12–13
  cytoskeletal networks, 14–16
  lipids, 13–14
  liquid-liquid phases, 11–12
  membrane proximal signaling, 14
SMACs, 2, 3f
synaptic cleft formation
  effector molecules, directed release of,
    23–24
  extracellular vesicles, 22–23
  membrane traffic, 21–22
TCR-p^{Ag}MHC interactions, 3–5
Immunoreceptor tyrosine-based activation
  motif (ITAM), 102
Immunoreceptor tyrosine-based inhibitory
  motifs (ITIM), 102
Inducible T-cell co-stimulator (ICOS), 8–9
Intercellular adhesion molecule-1 (ICAM-1),
  5–6, 12–13
Intramolecular signaling, antibodies, 154–157
Isothermal titration calorimetry (ITC),
  155–156, 158–160

J
Jurkat T cells, 18–19

K
Kaposi's sarcoma, 8–9
Killer cell lectin-like receptor G1 (KLRG1),
  114, 115f
Killer Ig-like receptors (KIRs), 101
  KIR3DL1-HLA-B*5701 complex, 108, 109f
  KIR2DL-HLA-C complexes, 106–108, 107f

L
Langerhan's cells, 8–9
Lattice light sheet (LLS) microscopy, 19–20
Leukocyte immunoglobulin-like receptors
  (LILRs), 101
  LILRB1-HLA-A2 complex, 108–109, 110f
  LILRB2-HLA-G complex, 108–109, 110f
  UL18-LILRB1 complex, 108–110, 110f
Linker of activated T cells (LAT), 10–11,
  13–14, 21–22
Lipids, 13–14
Low-resolution electron microscopy,
  153–154
Lupus erythematosus, anti-dsDNA antibodies.
  See Anti-dsDNA antibodies, SLE
Lymphocyte function associated 1 (LFA-1),
  5–6
Lymphocyte kinase (Lck), 9–11, 13–14
Ly49 receptors, 101
  Ly49H-m157 complex, 105–106, 106f
  MHC-I
    recognition, 102–104
    trans and *cis* interactions, 104–105, 105f

M
Major histocompatibility complex class I
  (MHC-I), 101
  KIR receptor, 101
    KIR3DL1-HLA-B*5701 complex, 108,
      109f
    KIR2DL-HLA-C complexes, 106–108,
      107f
  LILRs, 101
    LILRB1-HLA-A2 complex, 108–109, 110f
    LILRB2-HLA-G complex, 108–109, 110f
    UL18-LILRB1 complex, 108–110, 110f
  Ly49 receptors
    recognition, 102–104
    trans and *cis* interactions, 104–105, 105f
Maltose-binding protein (MBP), 90–91, 91f
Modular antibody model, 151–154
Monoclonal antibodies (mAbs). *See also*
      Synthetic antibody
  advantages, 82
  bispecific antibody, 82
  isolation of, 81–82
  research, diagnostic, and therapeutic
    reagents, 81–82
  therapeutic mAbs function, 82
Mouse cytomegalovirus (MCMV), 101, 105–106

N

Natural cytotoxicity receptors (NCRs), 101
  NKp30, 110–112, 112*f*
  NKp44 and NKp46, 110–111, 112*f*
Natural killer (NK) cell receptors, 101–102
  KLRG1, cadherin recognition, 114, 115*f*
  Ly49H-m157 complex, 105–106, 106*f*
  MHC-I recognition
    KIR receptor, 106–108
    LILRs, 108–110, 110*f*
    Ly49 receptors, 102–105, 105*f*
  NCRs, 101, 110–112, 112*f*
  NKG2A/CD94-HLA-E complex, 113*f*, 114
  NKG2D-MICA complex, 112–113, 113*f*
  NKp65-KACL complex, 115–116, 116*f*
Natural killer receptor domain (NKD),
  102–103
NCRs. *See* Natural cytotoxicity receptors (NCRs)
Nectins, 9
NKG2A/CD94-HLA-E complex, 113*f*, 114
NKG2D-MICA complex, 112–113, 113*f*
NK gene complex (NKC), 115–116, 116*f*
NKp65-KACL complex, 115–116, 116*f*
N-methyl-D-aspartate (NMDA) receptor, 138–139
Nuclear magnetic resonance (NMR), 42, 135,
  153

P

Paired immunoglobulin receptors (PIRs),
  108–109
pCons, 139
PD-1. *See* Programmed cell death 1 (PD-1)
Peripheral supramolecular activation cluster
  (pSMAC), 2, 3*f*
Phage display, synthetic antibodies
  antibody selection, 85, 87*f*
  design, 87–89, 89*f*
Phase separation, immunological synapses
  cell-cell interfaces, adhesion plane of, 12–13
  cytoskeletal networks, 14–16
  lipids, 13–14
  liquid-liquid phases, 11–12
  membrane proximal signaling, 14
Podosomes, 17–18
Point-mutant targeting antibodies, 94
Polyclonal antibodies (pAbs), 82
Posttranslational modification (PTM), 91*f*,
  94–95
Primary T cells, 18–19
Programmed cell death 1 (PD-1), 7–8, 66–69
Progressive multifocal leukoencephalopathy
  (PML), 94

R

R4A antibody, 136, 138–139

S

Secretory component (SC), 146–149
Secretory IgA (sIgA), 146–149
Signaling lymphocyte activation molecule
  (SLAM), 5–7
Single-chain Fv (scFv), 150
Single-domain antibodies (sdAbs), 150
Somatic hypermutations (SHMs), 84, 132,
  162–163
Super-resolution stimulated emission depletion
  (STED) microscopy, 19–20
Supported lipid bilayers (SLBs), 2, 12–13
Supramolecular activation clusters (SMACs),
  2, 3*f*
Surface plasmon resonance (SPR), 158–160
Synapses. *See* Immunological synapses
Synthetic antibody, 96
  applications
    conformation-specific antibodies, 90–91,
      91*f*
    cross-reactive antibodies, 92, 93*f*
    point-mutant targeting
      antibodies, 94
    PTMs, 91*f*, 94–95
  immunoglobulin structure and function,
    83–85, 83*f*
  phage-displayed antibody library
    antibody selection, 85, 87*f*
    design, 87–89, 89*f*
Systemic lupus erythematosus (SLE) related
  autoantibodies. *See* Anti-dsDNA
  antibodies, SLE

T

T-cell antigen receptor (TCR), 2. *See also*
  Immunological synapses
T-cells
  adhesion molecules and costimulatory
    receptors (*see* Cell-cell recognition)
  synapse (*see* Immunological synapses)
Total internal reflection fluorescence
  microscopy (TIRFM), 16–17
Tryptophan fluorescence, 131–132
"Two-in-one" antibody, 92, 93*f*

U

UL18-LILRB1 complex, 108–110, 110*f*

V

Vascular endothelial growth factor (VEGF), 92, 93*f*

Vasodilator-stimulated phosphoprotein (VASP) proteins, 16–17

W

Wiscott Aldrich syndrome protein (WASP), 3*f*, 14–19

X

X-ray crystallography, 106, 155–156
X-ray diffraction, 153

Y

Yeast display, 81–82

Z

Z-DNA-binding protein, 129
Zeta-associated kinase of 70 kDa (ZAP-70), 9–11

Printed in the United States
By Bookmasters